Manual of Fertility

Shikha Jain • Dattaprasad B. Inamdar

Editors

Manual of Fertility Enhancing Hysteroscopy

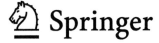 Springer

Editors
Shikha Jain
Director and Senior Consultant
Reproductive Medicine
Dreamz IVF
New Delhi
India

Dattaprasad B. Inamdar
Consultant Reproductive Medicine and
Assistant Professor (Dept of OBGY)
Bharati Vidyapeeth (Deemed to be
University) Medical College
Pune
Maharashtra
India

ISBN 978-981-10-8027-2   ISBN 978-981-10-8028-9   (eBook)
https://doi.org/10.1007/978-981-10-8028-9

Library of Congress Control Number: 2018937589

Printed on acid-free paper

This Springer imprint is published by the registered company Springer Nature Singapore Pte Ltd. part of
Springer Nature
The registered company address is: 152 Beach Road, #21-01/04 Gateway East, Singapore 189721,
Singapore

Foreword

Hysteroscopy is undoubtedly the beacon of modern gynecology, the golden idol revolutionizing one of the oldest branches of medicine. All aspiring gynecological surgeons are obligated to increase their knowledge and mastery of this minimally invasive technique which has provided solutions to countless pathologies of the female genital system. The diagnostic and concurrent therapeutic value of hysteroscopy lies in its ability to explore the female genital tract from the vagina up to and including the proximal salpinx. This edition pictorially illustrate the combined see and treat application of hysteroscopy while providing the necessary literature backing this majestic tool's value and efficacy. Ranging from office procedures to full-scale intrauterine surgery tackling uterine congenital anomalies, myomata, and adhesions, among others, there is no substitute for the magic stick of gynecology. This guide serves to set you on the road needed to grasp the ins and outs of office and operative hysteroscopy, and in doing so, the world of gynecology will be at your fingertips.

Cairo, Egypt   Osama Shawki
Giessen, Germany

Preface

"Hysteroscopy" is derived from the Greek words "hystera" (uterus) and "skopeo" (to view). Hysteroscopy is the visual examination of the cervix and interior of the uterus with an endoscope. Commander Pantaleoni performed the first hysteroscopy in 1869, but it was from 1970 onward when the rapid development in technology and instrumentation took place and the era of modern hysteroscopy evolved. Nowadays, hysteroscopy has become an essential tool to evaluate uterine cavity and to correct the abnormalities found within.

Though as a part of our training program we have read many excellent textbooks on hysteroscopy by the pioneers in the field, a book dedicated to its place in infertility management was a need of the time. Hence, the idea of this manual is to elaborate the diagnostic and therapeutic role of hysteroscopy specifically in the infertile women, without going into the details of other indications of gynecology and oncology. This book guides the reader through the basics of hysteroscopy with its instrumentation, indications, and contraindications and the choice of anesthesia along with the overview of complications. The authors have described different techniques of various operative procedures like polypectomy, myomectomy, adhesiolysis, and tubal cannulation in an easy to understand manner. It also gives insight on hysteroscopy in specific clinical conditions like mullerian anomalies, genital tuberculosis, ART, etc. Future applications are highlighted with the promising role of hysteroscopy in many new areas.

This manual is an illustrated yet comprehensive compilation by experts in the field of infertility, hysteroscopy, and assisted reproduction. We primarily aim this book at medical students and research fellows, but it would definitely help practicing gynecologists and ART specialists as well. The learning curve of hysteroscopy involves knowledge of the instruments and subject, hand-eye coordination, and clinical judgment. Salient features of this book are the following:

- Practical tips for performing diagnostic and operative hysteroscopy along with troubleshooting in difficult clinical situations.
- Updated with recent advances in the management of intrauterine pathologies interfering with natural or assisted conception.
- All the procedures are explained in a clear and precise text which is supported with latest evidence.

- Lucid illustration of diagnosis and management with tables, charts, and line diagrams.
- More than 100 high-magnification color photographs for better understanding of the pathology.

As a basic and quick reference guide, this book can be extremely valuable to budding hysteroscopic surgeons. We hope that the readers will find this manual helpful in optimizing their hysteroscopy skills resulting in improved patient care.

"What we know is what we see and what we see is what we treat."

New Delhi, India   Shikha Jain
Pune, India   Dattaprasad B. Inamdar

Acknowledgments

This book is dedicated to all our patients who have entrusted us. We are indebted to our authors who are all experts in the field of infertility. It's their generosity and efforts to put in practical experience and depth of knowledge together which has made this textbook a reality. We appreciate the constant support and encouragement of our family members. We pay our sincere thanks to Dr. Eti Dinesh and Springer Nature Publication for their invaluable help. Lastly, we are grateful to our teachers who guided us to this never-ending path of learning.

Shikha Jain
Dattaprasad B. Inamdar

Contents

About the Editors

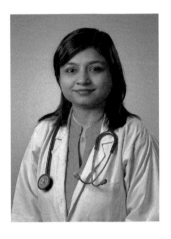

Shikha Jain, MBBS, MD, FNB (Rep Med), FICOG is the director and principal consultant in reproductive medicine at Dreamz IVF, New Delhi. She obtained her MBBS at the prestigious Sarojini Naidu Medical College, Agra, and her MD in Obstetrics and Gynaecology at Gandhi Medical College, Bhopal. She then completed her postdoctoral fellowship in reproductive medicine at the renowned Centre for Human Reproduction at Sir Ganga Ram Hospital, New Delhi. She topped all India levels in the fellowship exam conducted by the National Board of Examinations, India. She was the proud recipient of Dr. P. N. Wahi Gold Medal in 2002 and received first prize in the All India Quiz competition on infertility conducted by the Indian College of Obstetricians & Gynaecologists in 2011. She also won the best FNB student prize and the award for the best clinical paper presentation in 2013.

Dr. Shikha Jain is very active in clinical research. She has published a number of research papers in peer-reviewed journals and given clinical presentations on various aspects of infertility. She is a member of the teaching faculty for the advanced ART training programme and a peer reviewer on the board of the *International Journal of Fertility & Sterility*.

She is currently chair of IUI Committee of the Delhi chapter of the Indian Society of Assisted Reproduction (ISAR) and a member of Indian Fertility Society (IFS) special interest group on reproductive endocrinology. She is also a member of Infertility Committee of the Association of Obstetricians & Gynaecologists of Delhi (AOGD) and the Federation of Obstetric and Gynaecological Societies of India (FOGSI).

Her areas of expertise include reproductive medicine, fertility-enhancing gynaecological endoscopic surgeries and IVF. Her current interests focus on clinical trials to improve IVF outcome and fertility-preserving interventions in patients with cancer.

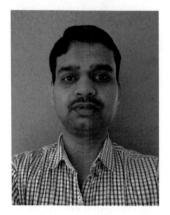

Dattaprasad B. Inamdar, MS, DNB, FNB (Rep Med) is currently working as an Assistant Professor in the Fertility Unit of the Department of Obstetrics and Gynaecology, Bharati Hospital, BVUMC, Pune. He pursued his postdoctoral fellowship in reproductive medicine at Sir Ganga Ram Hospital, New Delhi. He has a keen interest in research and recent advances in the field of infertility. His areas of expertise are assisted reproduction and fertility-enhancing gynaecological endoscopic surgeries.

List of Contributors

Aanchal Agarwal, DGO, DNB, FNB (Rep Med) Department of Infertility, IVF & Reproductive Medicine, B L K Superspeciality Hospital, New Delhi, India

Nameeta Mokashi Bhalerao, MBBS, MS (ObGy), DNB, FNB, PGDMLE Nova IVI Fertility services, Pune, India

Amitabh Dutta, MD Department of Anaesthesiology, Pain & Perioperative Medicine, Sir Ganga Ram Hospital, New Delhi, India

Shalu Gupta, MS, DNB, MNAMS, FNB IVF and Fertility, Cloud 9, Gurugram, Haryana, India

Shruti Gupta, MD (AIIMS), DNB, FNB Milann Kumarapark, Bengaluru, Karnataka, India

Parag Hitnalikar, MD (OBGY), FNB (Reprod Med) Orion Hospital, Pune, Maharashtra, India
Ruby Hall Clinic, Pune, Maharashtra, India

Dattaprasad B. Inamdar, MS, DNB, FNB (Rep Med) Department of Obstetrics and Gynecology, Bharati Vidyapeeth (Deemed to be University) Medical College, Pune, India

Shikha Jain, MBBS, MD, FNB (Rep Med), FICOG Dreamz IVF, New Delhi, India

Bimal John, MS, Dip. AES, Dip. MIS Credence Hospital, Trivandrum, Kerala, India

Mandeep Kaur, MD, FNB (Reprod. Med.) Nova IVI, Jalandhar, Punjab, India

Jyoti Mishra, MD (Obs & Gyn) Jaypee Hospital, Noida, UP, India

Ruma Satwik, DGO, DNB, FNB (Reprod Med) Centre of IVF and Human Reproduction, Institute of Obstetrics and Gynaecology, Sir Gangaram Hospital, New Delhi, India

Pinky Ronak Shah, DGO, DNB, FNB (Reprod Med) Morpheus Fertility Centre, Mumbai, Maharashtra, India

Sangita Sharma, MD (OBGY), DNB, FNB (Reprod Med) Manipal Fertility, Manipal Hospital, Jaipur, Rajasthan, India

Shilpa Sharma, DGO, DNB, MNAMS, FNB Aveya Natural IVF Fertility Centre, Delhi, India

Introduction and General Principles of Hysteroscopy

Mandeep Kaur and Bimal John

1.1 Introduction

The noun "hysteroscopy" is derived from the Greek words *hystera* (uterus) and *skopeo* (to view) [1]. Hysteroscopy is the visual examination of the cervix and interior of the uterus with an endoscope. Hysteroscopy is considered to be the "gold standard" method for evaluation of the uterine cavity [2]. However, hysteroscopy is invasive and costly, and therefore it is usually reserved for more detailed evaluation and treatment of abnormalities defined by noninvasive or less invasive methods.

Two-dimensional ultrasound is currently the first choice for basic, noninvasive evaluation of the uterine cavity [3]. Doubt of any intracavitary abnormalities such as a polyp, focal lesion, adhesions, myoma, developmental abnormality, retained products of conception, or any foreign body requires further evaluation. Although the use of office hysteroscopy as a first-line investigation in infertile couples is gaining popularity, there is lack of sufficient evidence to support it, especially if the ultrasound scan and hysterosalpingogram (HSG) are normal [4]. Other methods of cavity evaluation include three-dimensional ultrasonography (3D-USG), saline sonosalpingography (SSG), and magnetic resonance imaging (MRI).

The incidence of unsuspected abnormalities in the uterine cavity found by office hysteroscopy prior to IVF has been reported to be between 11% and 50%, with the risk increasing directly proportional to the number of failed in vitro fertilization (IVF) cycles [5–7]. It is also purported that hysteroscopy improves the outcome in IVF, especially in patients with history of implantation failure, if it is done immediately prior to the commencement of the IVF cycle [8]. This positive endometrial effect has been shown to be highest when hysteroscopy is performed up to 50 days prior to the embryo transfer [9]. Two mechanisms have been proposed for this

M. Kaur, MD, FNB (Reprod Med) (✉)
NOVA IVI, Jalandhar, Punjab, India

B. John, MS, Dip. A.E.S., Dip. M.I.S.
Credence Hospital, Trivandrum, Kerala, India

© Springer Nature Singapore Pte Ltd. 2018
S. Jain, D. B. Inamdar (eds.), *Manual of Fertility Enhancing Hysteroscopy*,
https://doi.org/10.1007/978-981-10-8028-9_1

beneficial effect—first, the ease of embryo transfers after hysteroscopy and, second, the higher implantation rates due to the stimulation or mechanical distension of the cavity.

Similarly, in patients with thin, refractory endometrium, hysteroscopy is considered to be the recommended investigation, as it has both diagnostic and therapeutic benefits. Hysteroscopy is also a useful modality in the work-up of patients with recurrent miscarriages due to higher chance of diagnosing a developmental defect [10]. However, hysteroscopy alone may be insufficient to treat uterine anomalies, as it requires additional confirmatory investigations such as a three-dimensional USG or MRI or a diagnostic laparoscopy.

Hysteroscopic removal of retained products of conception is also emerging as a superior method compared to simple dilatation and curettage, due to lower risk of adhesions as well as ensuring complete evacuation, thereby preserving future fertility [11]. With the advent of thinner and flexible endoscopes, office hysteroscopy is gaining popularity compared to conventional hysteroscopy, as it offers the benefit of minimal invasion along with shorter procedure time and lower complication rate.

1.2   Evolution of Modern Hysteroscopy

Philip Bozzini, known as the father of endoscopy, was the first to illuminate a cavity in the human body, when he used a telescope to visualize the inside of the urinary bladder [12]. In 1869, Commander Pantaleoni performed the first hysteroscopy on a postmenopausal woman, where he visualized a polyp and did chemical cauterization. Subsequently, Charles David developed an endoscope with a lamp behind a glass cover, allowing better visualization [13]. The choice of irrigation fluid also became a subject of debate, and initial use of sterile water had resulted in red cell hemolysis and renal failure.

Early work using fluids to distend the uterine cavity was published by C. J. Gauss in 1928, and later in 1934, C. Schroder reported that the ideal pressure required to distend the uterine cavity for good visibility without intratubal leak was around 30 mm of mercury [14]. Later, in 1947, the use of isotonic glucose solution as an irrigation fluid was reported by Creevy et al. [15].

From 1970 onward, there was rapid development of technology, which included the use of cold light instead of "hot" light through fiber-optic cables, replacement of thin lenses with thicker ones by Harold Hopkins [16], and also the use of carbon dioxide (CO_2) to distend the uterine cavity by Lindemann et al. [17]. By 1974, Karin Edstrom and Ingmar Fernstrom established the therapeutic use of hysteroscopy for lysis of adhesions and septal resection [18].

The development of the resectoscope, like most medical advancements, cannot be credited to a single scientist and has been attributed to three main discoveries: development of the incandescent lamp, high-frequency current, and the fenestrated sheath [19]. Maximilian Stern is credited to have first used the term "resectoscope" [20]. The resectoscope in its present form, which allows continuous irrigation, was devised by Iglesias et al. in 1975 [21].

As advances are being made in instrumentation and technology, the scope and application are also taking a leap, from simple, diagnostic procedures to technically challenging procedures such as the placement of Essure microinserts (Bayer HealthCare Pharmaceuticals Inc., Whippany, NJ) for sterilization and resection of scar and cervical ectopic pregnancies.

1.3   Preoperative Considerations

Careful planning for a hysteroscopic procedure is of utmost importance. Several aspects of hysteroscopy require the full understanding of the patient, and the surgeon needs to take her choices into consideration. Whether hysteroscopy should be performed in all infertile patients undergoing a diagnostic laparoscopy, especially in the presence of a normal HSG, is itself debatable. Other aspects such as the need and type of anesthesia, length of hospital stay, need for operative interventions during a diagnostic hysteroscopy, cost, etc. should be discussed, and the patient should be counselled accordingly. Needless to say, an informed consent needs to be obtained, with proper documentation of all possible complications related to the procedure and anesthesia.

Prophylactic antibiotic use is generally recommended to avoid postoperative infection, especially in operative hysteroscopy. The procedure is routinely performed in the follicular phase of the menstrual cycle, in order to prevent disruption of any undiagnosed pregnancy and also to avoid technical difficulties owing to overgrown endometrium in the luteal phase. Cervical ripening, for easier introduction of the scope and reducing the need for dilatation, is commonly achieved with the use of medications such as misoprostol (PGE1) and dinoprostone (PGE2) or with a laminaria tent. The mode of delivery during a previous pregnancy, parity, and estrogen status, etc. has variable effects on the outcome of these drugs. Misoprostol is preferred as it is stable at room temperature, cheap, and available in the tablet form and has tolerable, temporary, and dose-dependent side effects. Although misoprostol shows equal effectiveness whether administered orally, sublingually, or vaginally, the oral route is the most preferred route [22].

The traction of the cervix for easy insertion of the scope is one of the reasons for pain during office hysteroscopy. To avoid this, a vaginoscopic method has been propagated where the scope is introduced through the vagina and then under vision into the cervical canal, without any instrumentation. The pressure used for distension of the vagina is the same as that required for the uterine cavity distension, and there is no need to close the vulva, as the "weight" of fluid is sufficient to distend the vagina and provide visualization of the portio vaginalis.

1.4   Instrumentation

A thorough knowledge of instrumentation is essential in order to perform hysteroscopy. The basic requirements include an operating room with a camera unit and head, a light source with its cable for illumination, tools for distension of the uterine cavity, and the telescope with its sheath. Fluid management systems which maintain adequate and consistent intrauterine pressures are essential for operative procedures. The light source and camera head are no different from the ones used in the laparoscopic set up, needless to say that the camera should be of good resolution and supported with a quality light source. Panoramic view of the uterine cavity is possible only when there is adequate distension of the cavity, unlike contact hysteroscopy, which is less commonly performed nowadays.

A very organized operating room setup is essential for successful hysteroscopy. The entire team should be well versed with the equipments, and the instruments should be checked before use as well as on a periodic basis. A clear and unobstructed view of the video monitor that does not cause the surgeon's neck to strain is essential. A complete understanding of how to assemble the hysteroscope or resectoscope and its irrigation system is essential for smooth and safe surgery. The layout depends on the size of the OT and the preference of the surgeon (Fig. 1.1).

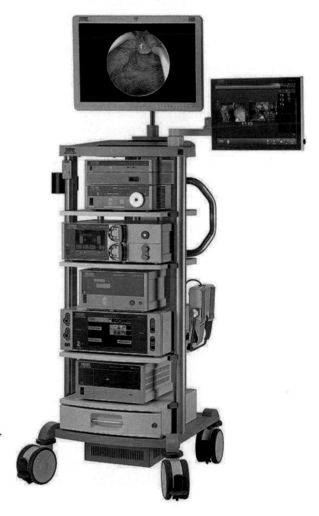

Fig. 1.1 Equipment cart for hysteroscopy, camera system, monitor, light source, fluid management device, electrosurgical unit, and documentation system (*Courtesy: Karl Storz*)

1.4.1 Camera and Monitor

The camera unit has a camera head, cable, and the camera control unit as its components. The lens on the camera is called a coupler, which magnifies the image to varying extents based on its capacity. It may be either fixed or detachable. The camera converts the optical image into an electrical image, sent via the cable to the processing unit and thereafter to the monitor, which reconverts this electrical signal to an optical image. Monitors display the image to the operator. To take full advantage of the increasing resolution of three-chip high-definition cameras, it is necessary to have supporting high-resolution medical monitors or high-definition TVs.

1.4.2 Light Source and Cord

Light sources generate light of different intensities and colors in order to illuminate the field of vision (Fig. 1.2). They may be Xenon- or Halogen bulb-based units or light-emitting diode (LED) units. Xenon bulbs generate higher intensity of light and last longer but are expensive. Light cord transmits the light from the source to the scope. Light cords are either fiber-optic or liquid-filled, and they disperse light equally across the diameter of the cord. The suitability of light source depends on the type of scope used, with powers ranging from 5 W LED to 300 W Xenon light sources. LED cold light sources have long operating life, and some models are battery operated and may not even require light cable.

1.4.3 Telescopes

A wide range of rod-lens telescopes are now available with various diameters and angles (Fig. 1.3). They range from 1.2 and 3 mm mini-telescopes to the 4 and 5 mm traditional telescopes. The angle of the lens may vary from 0, 12, 15, and 30°, giving a wide range of vision within the cavity. The acute angled telescopes (25, 30, and 45° angled lens), containing obliquely forward as opposed to a directly forward lens systems, are better suited for visualizing the uterine cornua and lateral walls. Having both 0–12° and 25–30° telescopes available for hysteroscopic and resectoscopic procedures gives the surgeon greater flexibility and confidence.

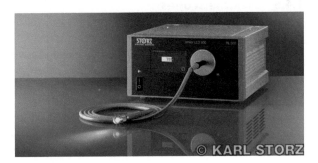

Fig. 1.2 Light source and cord (*Courtesy: Karl Storz*)

Fig. 1.3 Rigid telescope
(*Courtesy: Karl Storz*)

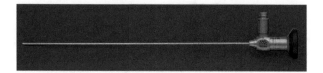

1.4.4 Sheaths

The sheaths that cover the telescopes provide protection as well as allow the passage of fluid or gas for distension and instruments for operative procedures (Fig. 1.4). There is usually an inner and outer fenestrated sheath, with space in between them for passage of the distension media. The inner sheath allows clean fluid into the cavity, while the outer fenestrated sheath helps to evacuate the fluid out of the cavity, thereby making it a continuous flow system. This double channel provides minimal inflow resistance with a slightly higher outflow resistance. This resulting continuous flow increases visibility while maintaining intrauterine pressure and distension. The instruments may be locked in place either by a rotary or twisting lock mechanism or with a snap-in connection type design.

Operating sheaths additionally have single or multiple working (operating) channels incorporated into the inner sheath. The combined outer diameter of newer instruments may be as low as 3.6 mm, and they may not require dilatation of the cervix. The operating channels allow the passage of 3–7 Fr caliber instruments such as scissors, graspers, electrocautery probes, etc. Sheaths with a single operating channel are thinner compared to the ones with a double operating channel for which the cervix may need dilatation, according to the maximum diameter of the assembled hysteroscope.

Smaller hysteroscopes have combined final diameters of the telescope with sheath that are efficient for diagnostic and office procedure. However, the field of view and brightness are reduced in smaller diameter scopes, and this can cause difficulty in a large uterine cavity or in the presence of bleeding or complicated pathologies. Telescopes with 4 mm diameter and outer sheaths of 7–8 mm containing multiple operating channels which allow 7 Fr caliber instruments are available to deal with such cases (Fig. 1.5). However, cervical dilatation is required as the maximum outer diameter in such cases may reach up to 9 mm.

1.4.5 Flexible Scopes

Newer scopes are flexible, providing good maneuverability that allows them to be bent according to alignment of the cervical canal and uterine cavity, usually without cervical dilatation. The diameter of the telescopes may be as small as 1.8 mm with outer diameters of 3.2 mm when combined with the sheath (Versascope, Gynecare, Ethicon Inc, Somerville, NJ). In case of extreme retroversion or anteversion of the uterus, such scopes allow atraumatic insertion. Flexible scopes also result in lower pain, especially in office hysteroscopy, but it may result in longer procedure time, higher maintenance cost, and lower resolution in comparison to the rigid scopes.

Fig. 1.4 Diagnostic sheath with a single inflow channel (*Courtesy: Karl Storz*)

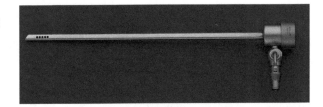

Fig. 1.5 Bettochi hysteroscope: telescope with sheaths (assembled) containing single working channel and fluid inlet and outlet ports (*Courtesy: Karl Storz*)

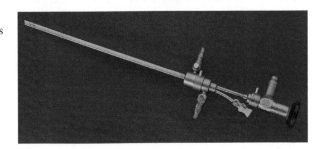

Fig. 1.6 Monopolar resectoscope with loop (*Courtesy: Karl Storz*)

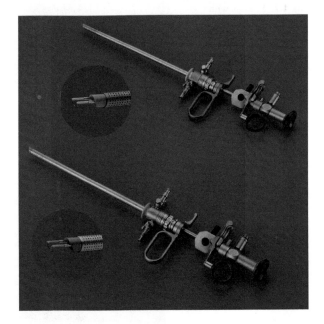

1.4.6   Resectoscopes

Gynecological resectoscopes are specialized operating hysteroscopes that allow the use of electrical energy within the uterine cavity in order to perform specialized procedures. They contain an electrode which works on a passive spring mechanism, which keeps it within the sheath in the neutral position, and allows advancing it beyond the sheath only during activation (Fig. 1.6).

1.4.7 Ancillary Instruments and Working Elements

Several instruments such as scissors, graspers, forceps, electroprobes, and catheters are now available for operative hysteroscopy, facilitating a wide range of surgical procedures (Figs. 1.7 and 1.8). They range from 3 to 7 Fr in diameter and can be passed through the operating channels in the sheath. They are mostly semirigid allowing manipulation without moving the scope. Extra care should be taken to insert these instruments under vision and keeping them under vision at all times of the surgery. Use of electroprobes mandates the same precautions taken during the use of electricity in any other surgical procedure. Nonelectrolyte solutions used to distend the uterine cavity, for use of monopolar energy sources, require extreme caution and monitoring to prevent complications such as fluid overload and electrolyte disturbances. Bipolar energy sources allow the use of electrolyte solutions which are comparatively safer.

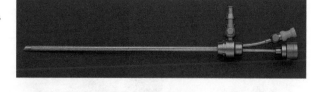

Fig. 1.7 Sheaths with working channel instruments size 5 Fr (*Courtesy: Karl Storz*)

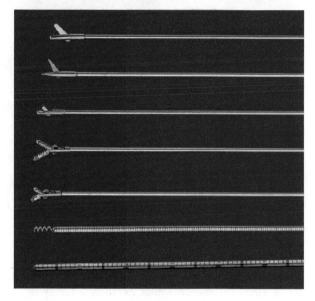

Fig. 1.8 Semirigid operating instruments (5 Fr) such as scissors, biopsy and grasping forceps, palpation probe, bipolar dissection electrode, and bipolar ball electrode (*Courtesy: Karl Storz*)

Fig. 1.9 Intrauterine
BIGATTI shaver
(*Courtesy: Karl Storz*)

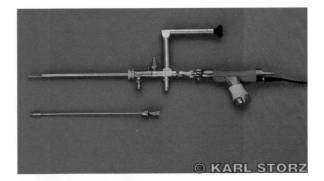

1.4.8 Morcellators

These are suction, mechanical or electrical energy-based, tubular cutting system developed to overcome disadvantages of the electrical energy-based resectoscopes (Fig. 1.9). On the basis of acknowledged limited information from the Review of the Manufacturer and User Facility Device Experience database, it is evident that although life-threatening complications such as fluid overload, uterine perforation, and bleeding occur less frequently, the data is limited and further research is recommended [23].

1.4.9 Laser Devices

Laser is used in hysteroscopic procedures as it is precise and can be used with electrolyte solutions. Various lasers such as the Nd-YAG, KTP-532, Argon, and tunable dye lasers have been used in treating different kinds of intrauterine conditions. However, its use is limited due to its technicality, cost implications, and the availability of bipolar energy-based resectoscopes.

1.4.10 Recording Devices

A wide array of devices for recording of both images and video are available now. Although they are optional, they are recommended from a medicolegal point of view. They aid in the process of patient counseling as well as serve as invaluable proof and documentation should any complication occur. Many surgeons also review their own videos, which helps in the process of research, learning, and refining skills. Record keeping is also important should a medicolegal case arise in the future. A multitude of compact systems for recording, transferring, printing, and storage are available commercially (Fig. 1.10).

Fig. 1.10 AIDA recording
system (*Courtesy Karl Storz*)

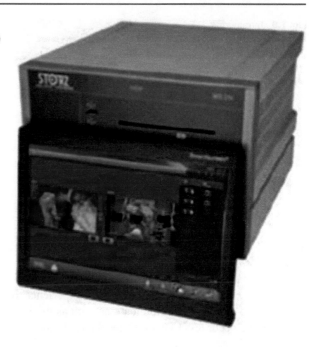

1.5   Distension Media

Panoramic view of the uterine cavity and the cervical canal need distension by a
transparent medium. Distension media could be either gas or liquid.

1.5.1   Gas Media

Carbon dioxide is the most commonly used gas medium, and it is relatively safe
since it is a product of the respiratory chain and easily absorbed. Its refractive index
is 1, essentially equivalent to air. However, care should be taken to restrict the flow
rate to <100 mL/min with the help of a special Hysteroflator, which has a maximum
flow rate of 100 mL/min. Most hysteroscopy examinations can be performed at a
flow rate of approximately 30–40 mL/min, with the intrauterine pressure at approximately 60–70 mmHg. Using a Laparoflator, which typically uses higher pressures
and flow rates that are suitable for laparoscopy, is dangerous as it increases the risk
of complications such as embolism and trauma.

1.5.2   Liquid Media

Liquid distension media-based hysteroscopy is preferred over gas-based hysteroscopy due to better visibility, less leakage through the tubes, less distortion of
the pathologies, lower glare of the light, and reduced risk of embolism. Liquid

media can be either electrolyte (lactated Ringer's or 0.45% and 0.9% normal saline solutions) or nonelectrolyte. Nonelectrolyte solutions may be either low-viscosity (glycine 1.5%, sorbitol 3%, or mannitol 5%) or high-viscosity (Hyskon high-molecular-weight dextran) fluids. An ideal medium should be isotonic, making it non-hemolytic and transparent, allowing ample visualization, and should be rapidly cleared from the body with no scope of toxicity or allergic reactions.

1.5.2.1 Aqueous Electrolyte Solutions

Aqueous Electrolyte Solutions such as physiological or 0.45% saline and lactated Ringer's are usually used for diagnostic hysteroscopy. Operative procedures using mechanical tools, laser, or bipolar current allow the use of such solutions. The presence of electrolytes in the media makes the procedure safer and reduces the risk of hyponatremia in case it is excessively absorbed. It is important to bear in mind that excessive absorption of saline (>1.5–2 L) may still produce pulmonary edema, and caution needs to be exercised.

1.5.2.2 Nonelectrolyte Solutions

Nonelectrolyte solutions with low viscosity, such as 1.5% glycine solution, 3% sorbitol, and 5% mannitol, and fluids with high viscosity, such as high-molecular-weight dextran, are used for operative hysteroscopy when monopolar electric current is required, since they are electrolyte-free. The quantity of fluid instilled and recovered should be carefully monitored and calculated in order to estimate the amount of fluid absorbed by the body, so that complications such as hyponatremia and other electrolyte imbalance can be prevented. Usually the acceptable fluid deficit should not be more than 1000–1500 mL in patients with normal cardiovascular function and not more than 750 mL in patients with compromised cardiovascular function. If the deficit crosses the safe limits, the procedure should be terminated and appropriate safety measures be taken immediately. Plastic pouches or modified drapes can be used to measure the output in low-resource settings where fluid management systems which automatically calculate such fluid deficits are not available. The factors affecting intravasation of liquid distension media are the intrauterine pressure, length of surgery, and the surface area of surgery.

A recent meta-analysis suggests that normal (0.9%) saline may be superior to CO_2 as a distension media in diagnostic hysteroscopy, although the authors recommend more randomized studies before guidelines can be formulated [24].

1.6   Fluid Management Systems

Uterine walls are thick and in apposition with each other, and therefore a positive pressure is required for its distension, unlike the urinary bladder which has thin, easily distensible walls. Moreover, the uterus is in direct communication with the peritoneal cavity through the fallopian tubes, and therefore leakage of fluid into the abdomen is possible.

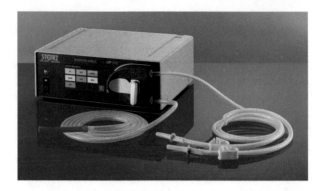

Fig. 1.11 Hamou Endomat fluid management system which can be used for both hysteroscopy and laparoscopy by changing the irrigation sets (*Courtesy: Karl Storz*)

Gravity is not sufficient to create the positive pressure required to distend the uterine cavity adequately, and mechanical pumps are required for the purpose. The pumps maintain constant intrauterine pressures by varying the distention fluid flow rate (Fig. 1.11). The goal is to use the lowest possible intrauterine pressure, which is around 40–80 mm of Hg in order to achieve adequate visualization of the uterine cavity. As the intrauterine pressure exceeds the mean arterial pressure, the risk of medium absorption increases. Newer devices measure the fluid pressure and the flow rate and allow limiting the intrauterine pressure. Higher filling pressures are associated with higher pain scores in office hysteroscopy, while lower filling pressures may affect the visibility. These systems are costly, but they allow uterine distension in a controlled manner, especially for operative procedures.

1.7   Electrosurgery in Hysteroscopy

Innovations over the last several decades, such as newer generators, return electrode monitoring, specialized electrodes, etc., have dramatically increased the efficacy and safety of electrosurgery in hysteroscopy. Two types of circuits are routinely employed for surgeries. In the monopolar circuit, current passes from the generator to an active electrode and returns from the surgical site through the patient. However, in a bipolar circuit, there is a return electrode adjacent to the active electrode which facilitates current flow without any major flow of current through the patient.

The relative non-conductive nature of the distension media increases impedance, which necessitates a high voltage for initiation. Hence, the electrosurgical units require a higher peak voltage, and the surgeon and assistant should be well-versed with the electrosurgical unit settings needed for various operative hysteroscopic procedures.

1.7.1   Monopolar Currents

Monopolar currents generated by high-frequency generators can be used for cutting and coagulation (Fig. 1.12). In order to avoid damage to the adjacent organs, the lowest possible power settings are recommended.

Fig. 1.12 Monopolar and bipolar generator (*Courtesy Karl Storz*)

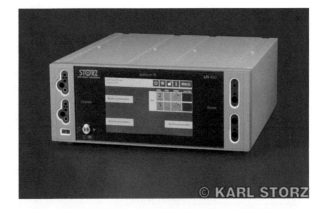

Fig. 1.13 Bipolar resectoscopes (*Courtesy: Karl Storz*)

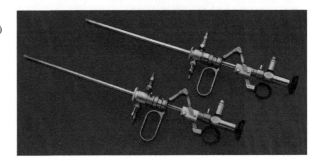

1.7.2 Bipolar Energy

Bipolar energy-based resectoscopes became available only more recently (Fig. 1.13). They can be used with electrolyte solutions making them much safer [25]. The bipolar system consists of a bipolar electrical generator and electrodes of various types which provide controlled tissue removal by vaporization. Each electrode has an active point at the tip and a return electrode at the shaft, and therefore, collateral damage is very minimal.

1.8 Sterilization

After use, the telescope, sheath, and the instruments need to be rinsed, washed, and dried thoroughly with care especially while cleaning the internal channels. Ancillary instruments are extremely fragile and delicate and therefore require great attention during cleaning. Sterilization of the instruments can be done using glutaraldehyde (>2.4% concentration, for at least 10 h), which is the most commonly used technique as it is cheap and easily available, overnight gas ethylene oxide (ETO) sterilization (at least for 15 h), or hydrogen gas plasma (50 min cycles). All microorganisms and spores are destroyed by these methods.

Table 1.1 Comparison of the commonly used sterilization methods

Method	Benefits	Drawbacks
Steam	– Nontoxic – Penetrates lumens – Rapid cycle time	– Not for heat-sensitive instruments – May induce rust – Microsurgical instruments get damaged with repeated exposure
Hydrogen peroxide gas plasma	– Shortest cycle time – Best for heat-sensitive equipment – Equipment is easy to install and monitor and uses electrical outlet only – No aeration time – Leaves no tissue residue – Environment friendly	– Linens cannot be processed – Restrictions based on length and diameter of equipments – Requires synthetic packaging – Small chamber size
Glutaraldehyde	– Numerous studies on its use – Compatible with most materials – Inexpensive	– Slow microbicidal activity – Pungent and irritating odor – Coagulates blood and fixes tissue to surface
ETO gas sterilization	– Penetrates lumens – Easy to install – Compatible with most medical equipment	– Toxic, inflammable, and carcinogenic – Aeration time to remove residue – Lengthy cycle – Small chamber size

Most metallic parts can be autoclaved, but telescopes and plastic-coated parts cannot be autoclaved. Telescopes need to be handled with care, and one should avoid dropping and bending of instruments during sterilization. After removing from the chemical disinfectant, using the recommended duration and concentration, the scopes need to be rinsed with sterile water, dried, and then stored. In between two procedures, disinfection of the scopes can be done by immersion in glutaraldehyde (>2% concentration, for a minimum of 20–45 min). The drawback is that bacterial spores are not destroyed. A comparison of the most commonly employed methods of sterilization is given in the table below (Table 1.1).

1.9   Training

Although diagnostic hysteroscopy is relatively safe, operative hysteroscopic procedures should be performed in well-equipped operating rooms, by experienced operators in order to reduce the risk of complications. Since very few academic programs for ObGyn residents incorporate hysteroscopic training in their curriculum, most of the practicing gynecologists rely on short programs for acquiring skills, leaving room for complications when complex surgeries are attempted.

A variety of surgical simulators and training devices are available to assist surgeons in learning and practicing the technical skills needed for conducting hysteroscopy. Virtual reality simulators are limited by their cost. It is also important to understand the assembly/disassembly of equipment, basic principles of electrosurgery, as well as the principles related to the safe use of distension media.

Table 1.2 Levels of training based on hysteroscopic operations

Level 1	Diagnostic hysteroscopy and targeted biopsy
	Removal of simple polyps
	Removal of intrauterine contraceptive devices
Level 2	Proximal fallopian tube cannulation
	Division of minor uterine synechiae
	Removal of pedunculated myomas
Level 3	Uterine septum resection
	Endometrial resection/ablation
	Resection of submucous/intramural myoma
	Division of major uterine synechiae
	Operative procedures such as lysis of severe synechiae, complete septal resection, and removal of myomas with intramural extension

Three levels of hysteroscopy training are described, based on the complexity of the procedure and skill required (Table 1.2) [26].

Key Points

1. Hysteroscopy has evolved into a gold standard technique for visualization and treatment of all intracavitary abnormalities.
2. Cervical ripening with misoprostol allows easy insertion of scopes in office hysteroscopies.
3. Normal saline is preferable to carbon dioxide as a distension medium.
4. Electrolyte solutions are safer but allow electrosurgery with bipolar energy source only.
5. Adequate distension and visualization of uterine cavity occurs with intrauterine pressures ranging from 40 to 80 mm of mercury, and intrauterine pressure should not increase beyond the mean arterial pressure.
6. Monopolar resectoscopes need nonelectrolyte solutions as well as vigilance on fluid deficit.
7. Hysteroscopic morcellators have a significant learning curve for regular usage.
8. Fluid management systems allow cavity distension in a controlled manner, especially for operative hysteroscopies.
9. Glutaraldehyde is the most commonly used, and hydrogen peroxide gas plasma is the best method for sterilization of equipment.
10. Hysteroscopic operative procedures need a good level of training and should not be attempted by inexperienced surgeons.

References

1. Gauss CJ. Hysteroskopie. Arch Gynaecol. 1928;133:18.
2. Bozdag G, Aksan G, Esinler I, Yarali H. What is the role of office hysteroscopy in women with failed IVF cycles? Reprod Biomed Online. 2008;17:410–5.
3. Ragni G, Diaferia D, Vegetti W, Colombo W, Arnoldi M, Crosignani PG. Effectiveness of sono-hysterography in infertile patient work up: a comparison with transvaginal ultrasonography and hysteroscopy. Gynaecol Obstet. 2005;59:184–8.

4. Crosignani PG, Rubin BL. Optimal use of infertility diagnostic tests and treatments. The ESHRE Capri Workshop Group. Hum Reprod. 2000;15:1723–32.
5. Fatemi HM, Kasius JC, Timmermans A, et al. Prevalence of unsuspected uterine cavity abnormalities diagnosed by office hysteroscopy prior to in vitro fertilization. Hum Reprod. 2010;25:1959–65.
6. Levi-Setti PE, Colombo GV, Savasi V, et al. Implantation failure in assisted reproduction technology and a critical approach to treatment. Ann N Y Acad Sci. 2004;1034:184–99.
7. Elter K, Yildizhan B, Suntay T, Kavak ZN. Diagnostic hysteroscopy before IVF: which women are candidates? J Turkish German Gynaec Assoc. 2005;6:217–9.
8. Pundir J, Pundir V, Omanwa K, et al. Hysteroscopy prior to the first IVF cycle: a systematic review and meta-analysis. Reprod Biomed Online. 2014;28:151–61.
9. Karyalcin R, et al. Office hysteroscopy improves pregnancy rates following IVF. Reprod Biomed Online. 2012;25:261–6.
10. Weiss A, Shalev E, Romano S. Hysteroscopy may be justified after two miscarriages. Hum Reprod. 2005;20(9):2628–31.
11. Hooker AB, et al. Long term complications and reproductive outcome after the management of retained products of conception: a systematic review. Fertil Steril. 2016;105:156–64.
12. Engel RME. Philipp Bozzini-The Father of Endoscopy. J Endourol. 2004;17(10):859–62.
13. Valle RF. Development of hysteroscopy: from a dream to a reality, and its linkage to the present and future. J Minim Invasive Gynecol. 2007;14(4):407–18.
14. Schroeder C. Uber den Ausbau and die Leistungun der Hysteroskopie. Arch Gynakol. 1934;156:407.
15. Creevy CD, Webb EA. A fatal hemolytic reaction following transurethral resection of the prostate gland: a discussion of its prevention and treatment. Surgery. 1947;21:56–66.
16. Gow JG. Harold Hopkins and optical systems for urology-an appreciation. Urology. 1998;52:152–7.
17. Lindemann HJ. Historical aspects of hysteroscopy. Fertil Steril. 1973;24:230.
18. Edström KGB. Intrauterine surgical procedures during hysteroscopy. Endoscopy. 1974;6(03):175–81.
19. Nesbit RM. A history of transurethral prostatic resection. In: Silber SJ, editor. Transurethral resection. New York, NY: Appleton-Century-Crofts; 1977. p. 1–17.
20. Stern M. Resection of obstructions at the vesical orifice. JAMA. 1926;87:1726–30.
21. Iglesias JJ, Sporer A, Gellman AC, et al. New Iglesias resectoscope with continuous irrigation, simultaneous suction, and low intravesical pressure. J Urol. 1975;114:929–33.
22. Song T, et al. Effectiveness of different routes of misoprostol administration before operative hysteroscopy: a randomised controlled trial. Fertil Steril. 2014;102:519–24.
23. Haber K, et al. Hysteroscopic morcellation: review of the manufacturer and user facility device experience (MAUDE) database. J Minim Invasive Gynecol. 2015;22(1):110–4.
24. Craciunas L, et al. Carbon dioxide vs normal saline as distension medium for diagnostic hysteroscopy: systematic review of randomised controlled trials. Fertil Steril. 2013;100:1709–14.
25. Fernandez H, et al. Operative hysteroscopy for infertility using normal saline solution using co-axial bipolar electrode. A pilot study. Hum Reprod. 2000;15(8):1773–5.
26. Gordon AG. Safety and training. Baillieres Clin Obstet Gynaecol. 1995;9(2):241–9.

Anesthesia for Hysteroscopy

2

Amitabh Dutta

Hysteroscopy is an essential intervention dealing with surgical, diagnostic, and procedural management of gynecology and fertility sciences. With continuous development, hysteroscopy, an otherwise minor procedure, has evolved considerably, and now its indications include an expansive mandate (Table 2.1) [1, 2]. Though generally a short-duration procedure, hysteroscopy intervention is as contentious and complex as it may be, especially on account of the intended outcome as well as the anesthetic implications therein. Over and above the procedural intricacies of the operation, anesthesia management of hysteroscopy subsumes equal importance and must be approached in a methodical manner [3].

2.1 Anesthesia Management for Hysteroscopy

Per se, a hysteroscopy procedure can be undertaken under any kind of anesthesia, i.e., general anesthesia (GA) or local anesthesia (LA), or a range of central neuraxial blockade options. While an understanding and non-anxious patient may agree to hysteroscopy under pharmacologic sedation and LA administered by the gynecologist, majority prefers a GA technique to ward off fear, procedure-related pain, and stress due to anticipation of the expected outcome; to cope with alien operating room (OR) environment; and to sleep through the procedure. Irrespective of the anesthesia type the patient opts for, there are several implications that need specific attention [3, 4].

A. Dutta, MD
Senior Consultant and Professor, Department of Anaesthesiology, Pain and Perioperative Medicine, Sir Ganga Ram Hospital, Ganga Ram Institute for Medical Education and Research (GRIPMER), New Delhi, India

Member, Ethics Committee and Science (Protocol) Committee, Sir Ganga Ram Hospital, Ganga Ram Institute for Medical Education and Research (GRIPMER), New Delhi, India

© Springer Nature Singapore Pte Ltd. 2018
S. Jain, D. B. Inamdar (eds.), *Manual of Fertility Enhancing Hysteroscopy*,
https://doi.org/10.1007/978-981-10-8028-9_2

Table 2.1 Indications for hysteroscopy

Operative hysteroscopy
Polyps, fibroid excision
Adhesiolysis/Asherman syndrome
Endometrial ablation/biopsy
Uterine septum resection
Diagnostic hysteroscopy
Analysis of uterine lining
Assessment of abnormal bleeding
Identification of the septum, malformed uterus
Hysteroscopy for specialized Intervention
Evaluation for in vitro fertilization (IVF)
Fallopian tube morphology analysis
Emergency hysteroscopy
Unaccounted bleeding per vagina/polymenorrhea

2.1.1 Implications Due to Patient Factors

2.1.1.1 Preoperative Preparation and Fasting Status Management

Typically, hysteroscopy procedures are listed on the forenoon list on a day care basis. Patients are advised to come in the morning directly from the home on an empty stomach. These procedures are performed early in the day so as to avoid uncomfortable situations, such as over-fasting, dissatisfaction with prolonged wait for a small procedure, hypoglycemia and electrolyte imbalance, the problems of unscheduled overstay, and delayed hospital discharge.

General preparation includes antianxiety medication in the morning of surgery, and continuing on with regular treatment, the patient may be prescribed for coexistent medical problems. The patient posted for surgery the next morning ought to be fasted for hysteroscopy and anesthesia. Despite abundance of prevailing fasting guidelines [5, 6], more or less, a patient electively posted for surgery must be adequately fasted to solid food intake (6 h or more), liquids (more than 4 h), and clear fluids (3 h). Patients who visit hospital for hysteroscopy on a day-case basis should be advised to come to the hospital in time to avoid difficulties arising out of hunger due to unaccustomed over-fasting, anxiety, hemodynamic over-response to anesthetics, acidity, and having to go back home late in the evening.

2.1.1.2 Coexisting Illness(s)

Patients undergoing hysteroscopy may range from young adults to elderly females. Any patient may be in receipt of medication(s) for comorbidities other than the hysteroscopy indication itself. Patients belonging to the older age group, especially around menopause, may have an associated systemic medical illness that can influence anesthesia and/or the outcome of hysteroscopic evaluation/intervention. Therefore, proactive management and optimization of coexisting systemic illness before receiving anesthesia and undergoing hysteroscopy are keys to positive/

intended outcome [6]. The most common diseases that afflict women of this age group (40–80 years) are hypertension, diabetes, and hypothyroidism, in that order. The hypertensive patients on prescription treatment should be advised to take morning dose of antihypertensive(s) to avoid intervention-related hypertensive response and possible increase in surgical bleeding that hampers endoscopic visualization and the hysteroscopy management. Patients who are incidentally detected with increased blood pressure for the first time or those who have an erratic history of drug consumption should be reevaluated. Those with presence of other systemic disease as well or are of old age should proceed to specific cardiology evaluation along with other specialty consultation if required. Patients with diabetes mellitus should undergo careful preanesthetic evaluation with the most recent reports detailing the metabolic profile (fasting, random, and fasting blood sugar; glycosylated hemoglobin). The anesthesiologist should refer them to dedicated endocrinologist for further assessment in case of blood sugar non-control, adverse metabolic status, and sign/symptoms of osmotic derangement like polyphagia, polyuria, or polydipsia. The diabetic patients and their attendants should be advised to reach the OR early on the day of surgery, and preferably get the hysteroscopy done as a first case, so as to resume oral intake early after the surgery is over. Patients are to be strictly advised to omit/stop the morning dose of oral hypoglycemic agents in order to decrease the likelihood of unanticipated/precipitant fall in the normal blood sugar levels in the perioperative period. For those afflicted with hypothyroidism, the patient may be advised to take the morning dose of supplemental thyroid drugs. In all of the aforementioned diseases, the patient should present them to anesthesiologist with a complete battery of the most recent laboratory test reports (within a month of surgery) and communicate clearly about the history and current control. Recently, the problem of obesity has become common among patients of the younger age group coming for hysteroscopy. Commonly, the obesity is associated with any of the above metabolic or endocrinology ailment. Patients with obesity may require acute attention for they pose problems during anesthesia, positioning for hysteroscopy, and recovery. A thorough assessment is required to identify the presence of obstructive sleep apnea (OSA). If OSA is present, appropriate measures are proactively taken in order to avoid problems that delay postoperative recovery. Over and above the uncontrolled systemic diseases the patient may be having, absolute contraindications for hysteroscopy should always be considered (Table 2.2).

In view of the above stated, the choice of anesthesia technique and application approach needs to be individualized on a case-to-case basis.

Table 2.2 Contraindications for hysteroscopy	• Patient refusal
	• Active/ongoing infection
	• Allergic to irrigation fluid
	• Acute pelvic trauma
	• Advanced cancer (endometrial, cervical, uterine, fallopian tube)

2.1.2   Implications Specific to Anesthesia Management

2.1.2.1 Choice of Anesthesia

The management of anesthesia depends greatly on the indication for which hysteroscopy is being planned. While a general "SAFE" (short-acting drugs and fast emergence) approach to anesthesia is highly desirable, appropriate selection of anesthesia technique is important for patient safety and quality-of-anesthesia care.

On one hand, for diagnostic hysteroscopy, where the only problematic step during the procedure comprises of dilatation of cervix and the passage of hysteroscope into the uterine cavity, usually, a balanced combination of pharmacological sedation [7] and local analgesia (e.g., trans-cervical lidocaine instillation) [8] suffices. A typical analgo-sedation regimen for outpatient anesthesia for hysteroscopy includes intravenous fentanyl 1–2 μg/kg followed by short-acting benzodiazepine midazolam 0.5–1.0 mg. It is to be noted that that order is followed; otherwise if the patient is administered midazolam first, there is a likelihood of uncomfortable dysphoria. On the other hand, even for diagnostic utero-endoscopy in patients with infertility, full general anesthesia (GA) is advised in order to achieve accuracy with the technique and for helping the pent-up and anxious females who are already constrained with the burden of successful outcome. In case of hysteroscopy procedure that involves operative intervention, such as polypectomy, endometrial biopsy, adhesiolysis, or when hysteroscopy is combined with laparoscopy, a run-of-the-mill endotracheal GA is instituted. Hysteroscopy is usually a short procedure, and hence short-acting drugs are employed for GA such that they get eliminated rapidly and the patient becomes discharge-ready and street fit early. Propofol-based total intravenous anesthesia (TIVA) technique is commonly employed without the use of any neuromuscular blockade. A standardized routine for administering GA for hysteroscopy involves, in this order: fentanyl citrate 1–2 μg/kg, induction of anesthesia with propofol 1.5–2.5 mg/kg, and maintenance of anesthesia with either inhalation technique (sevoflurane/desflurane in oxygen-air mixture) or propofol infusion (TIVA technique) titrated to keep adequate anesthesia depth as measured with EEG-based monitoring system (e.g., bispectral index monitoring). If the operative hysteroscopy is anticipated to be of long duration or requires the patient to be absolutely still for fine surgical manipulations, then a relaxant is administered. Atracurium besylate (0.5 mg/kg), a short-acting skeletal muscle relaxant, is preferred for the above stated purpose.

Central neuraxial anesthesia, including spinal anesthesia, an epidural, or a combined spinal-epidural block, can be considered as sole anesthesia option for patients who refuse to consent for either LA or GA and have coexisting systemic illness that precludes administration of GA and in emergency situation when the patients are not adequately fasted to receive GA safely. However, two important aspects have to be settled before opting for neuraxial blocks, i.e., the patient should not be having preexistent clinical dysautonomia that brings about wide fluctuations in blood pressure and preferably possess intact coagulation profile (normal bleeding/clotting time). Spinal anesthesia is the preferred neuraxial technique employed for hysteroscopy procedure, and the LA drug (bupivacaine heavy 0.5%) has to be used selectively (5–10 mg with or without fentanyl 20–25 μg) to ensure adequate level of sensory analgesia and also to gain quick recovery [9]. It is important to bear in mind that for both adequate intensity of spinal block effect in the pelvic region of interest to the gynecologist and hemodynamic stability during the hysteroscopy procedure, the spinal should be administered in sitting position. Common problems following spinal anesthesia, such as post-dural puncture headache [10], lower limb paresthesia, and neck stiffness, must be explained to the patient at the time of obtaining informed consent. In case these complications are present, the patient should be reassured and the problem managed as per related guidelines.

The use of LA drugs (bupivacaine, ropivacaine, lidocaine) should be avoided in patients with a history of known allergy. Even when used for surface anesthesia of for spinal anesthesia, the LA drug allergy and its catastrophic events must be kept in mind, and the standby emergent care kept ready. Ideally, each episode of LA drug administration should be preceded by allergy elicitation tests.

2.1.2.2 Airway Management

Whenever GA technique is selected for a hysteroscopy intervention, it is imperative to use an airway conduit that is safe and does not interfere with hysteroscopy itself or the post-procedure patient recovery. It is advisable to use endotracheal anesthesia always because of the safety and consistency of performance it proffers. However, due to advent of an array of supraglottic airway devices, such as laryngeal mask airways (LMA: ProSeal, Classic, I-gel, Baska), which are propagated for its utility in decreasing postoperative sore throat, are easy to place and remove, do not need that much expertise, and are disposable, many centers have modified their guidelines to include them in the armamentarium on a regular basis. However, the author is wary of its potential for lack of safety on account of inability to preclude pulmonary aspiration of gastric contents. Also, when compared to endotracheal tube airway control, the supraglottic airway devices are often inconsistent in terms of intraoperative mechanical ventilation performance. Sometimes, for a very short hysteroscopy procedure, inhalation GA can be administered for an adequately fasted patient with a fitting facemask as airway conduit. One must always remember though, in any case, the anesthesiologist should be trained and experienced to gain control with full GA with tracheal intubation.

2.1.3   Implications Arising Out of Hysteroscopy Procedure

2.1.3.1 Patient Positioning for Hysteroscopy

Typically, the patient undergoing hysteroscopy needs to be positioned in lithotomy/extended lithotomy position so as to facilitate access to the pelvis and conduction of hysteroscopy [11]. Lithotomy position, an apparently easy position to achieve once the patient is under GA, has its own share of problems: like, nerve damage/stretch neuropraxia (posterior tibial nerve, popliteal nerve, and lateral cutaneous nerve of thigh), pressure sores (gluteal, sacral, thigh), deep vein thrombosis, and postoperative sacroiliac and back pain. Therefore, diligent patient positioning is an absolute prerequisite before hysteroscopy can even begin. Appropriate padding of pressure sites, such as under the knee, calves, buttocks, and ankles, is the key to avoid uncalled problems. In case neuropraxia or peripheral neuropathy has happened, a thorough neurologic evaluation, pharmacologic management, and postsurgery rehabilitative physiotherapy are required till adequate recovery is attained. An important add-on to placing the patient in lithotomy position is that, not uncommonly, they are also made to position in Trendelenburg or the reverse-Trendelenburg position. If that is the case, the complete gamete of physiologic implications of positioning becomes active and must be handled with extraordinary care.

2.1.3.2 Intrauterine Space Creation for Endoscopic/Surgical Instrument Manipulations

Often, continuous intrauterine irrigation with fluid is utilized to open up the uterine space, to improve overall vision, and to facilitate diagnostic and operative actions of the gynecologist. Different types of fluids are used (Table 2.3), which are selected

Table 2.3 Distending media for hysteroscopy [12]

Media	Advantages	Disadvantages
Gaseous		
• Carbon dioxide (CO_2) [13]	• Almost none	• Frequent blockade of endo-vision by blood/endometrial debris • Low volume CO_2 can induce cardiovascular collapse • Requires special insufflation unit • Can be used for diagnostic hysteroscopy only • Postoperative pain, vasovagal episodes
Fluids		
• High-viscosity fluid [14] (e.g., 32% dextrose 70 in 10% glucose)	• Immiscible with blood • Allows uterine cavity evaluation even in presence of bleeding	• Hyperosmolar, cannot use volume >300 mL • Propensity for fluid overload high • Tendency to "caramelize" on equipment leading to damage, precludes use with flexible hysteroscope • Anaphylaxis with dextran 70 not uncommon (incidence 1:821) [15]
• Low viscosity fluids		

• Electrolyte-free
  3% sorbitol
  1.5% glycerine
  5% mannitol
  3% sorbitol + 0.5% mannitol
	• Excellent visibility	• Reduction in serum osmolality
		• Hyponatremia by osmotic diuresis
		• Hyperammonemia with CNS consequences

• Electrolyte Plus 0.9% normal saline [13]	• Isotonic media • Does not lead to hyponatremia • Can use bipolar energy system	• Not suitable for use of energized monopolar cautery radiofrequency generator system

on the basis of the electrolyte content, osmolality, and viscosity [12]. It is essential that an electrolyte-free irrigation fluid be used for surgical hysteroscopy. It is also to be noted that high driving pressures (80–150 mmHg) are necessary to distend the thick-walled uterus [3]. Distending media can either be gas (CO_2) or fluid.

It is very important that the anesthesiologist be wary of the type of fluid, volume/rate of fluid in the intrauterine cavity at the time of hysteroscopy, and intrauterine pressure created due to fluid irrigation. As a rule, the set limits for parameters indicating safety of irrigation fluid management should be adhered to. Most importantly, the patient should be closely monitored for any hemodynamic change (in case of GA), alteration in neurologic status (if the patient is under LA or spinal anesthesia) to detect uterine perforation early. Finally, the temperature of the irrigation fluid must be kept close to the body temperature lest it may cause hypothermia and delayed recovery (if the fluid is cold) or uterine mucosa burn (in case the fluid warmer than body temperature). Further, the anesthesiologist should be prepared to manage (1) fluid overload-induced pulmonary edema, (2) hypothermia, and (3) dys-electrolytemia. In view of the above, all throughout the hysteroscopy procedure, communication with the operating gynecologist becomes very important so as to avoid or intervene early.

2.1.3.3 Managing Endoscopic Vision Inside the Uterus

Maintenance of a clear endoscopic vision is vital to efficient and effective hysteroscopic manipulation. Many methods are used but have their own problems. If hot water is used to clean the distal scope lens, then one should be careful that upon reentry, the hot tip can cause trauma to the uterine mucosa. If glutaraldehyde solution is used, then allergic consequences should be kept in mind. Irrigation fluid should be turned over continuously, especially during surgical hysteroscopy.

2.1.3.4 Use of Energized Equipment

Modern-day resectoscopes are endo-luminal surgical systems comprsing of an endoscope, an inflow/outflow sheath for irrigation fluid, and an interface electrode that is connected to a electrosurgical/radiofrequency generator. Whereas a monopolar RF system is not compliant with electrolyte irrigation solutions as they conduct electricity, bipolar RF systems are costly and not in common use [16]. Operative hysteroscopy involves the use of a host of energized-tip equipment to facilitate cutting and coagulation. In this regard, the anesthesiologist must be aware of the electrical safety issues with the use of such devices and take preparatory actions to prevent them.

2.1.3.5 Management of Combined Hysteroscopy-Laparoscopy

Not uncommonly, the patients undergo laparoscopy and hysteroscopic evaluation together, especially in infertility cases. While the laparoscopic vision enables physicians to note the dye-spill form the fallopian tubes to assess patency, the hysteroscopic assessment helps one to categorize fibroids of the uterus more accurately. In either case, decision for corrective action can be taken more effectively. When combined hysteroscopy and laparoscopy are undertaken, the anesthesiologist should take appropriate care to entertain implications of carbo-peritoneum and intrauterine irrigation on patients' physiology.

2.2   Complications of Hysteroscopy [17, 18]

2.2.1   Intrauterine Bleeding

Largely, hysteroscopy is a minor procedure that does not lead to major bleeding. However, since the uterus is a well-perfused organ, during operative resection of endometrium and deeper layers, there is a likelihood of opening up of venous sinuses and active arterial bleeders. Operative hysteroscopy may result in bleeding that does not always require a counterresponse (e.g., transfusion of blood) and may still pose problem. First, there may be difficult-to-maintain endoscopic vision-hampering surgery; second, active bleeding, which attains significance under magnified endoscopic vision, can create panic among the gynecologists who then resort to unscrupulous actions resulting in more trauma and excessive use of energized-tip equipment. Both of them are a perfect recipe for disaster that may include more bleeding, uterine perforation, uncalled blood transfusion, etc. Typically, bleeding during operative hysteroscopy can be contained by waiting, stopping irrigation, and applying mechanical plugs (gel-foam, surgical, fibrillar filaments) and pharmacologic antibleeding agents (e.g., tranexamic acid) [19]. The operating gynecologist should lower the irrigation pressure, so that active bleeders can be identified and coagulated.

2.2.2   Uterine Perforation

The incidence of uterine wall perforation during hysteroscopy is 0.8% [20]. Hysteroscopy by itself is a procedure that requires careful and focused conduct. Perforation of uterine wall can happen due to mechanical perforation with the instrument/endoscope, increased irrigation fluid pressure, overzealous attempts for thick biopsy specimen retrieval, overzealous attempts to remove a large myoma and, sometimes, going through a wall defect taking it to be fallopian tube opening. Since the weakest part of uterus is the fundus, perforation most commonly occurs at fundal site. If the operating gynecologist sees a yellow hue during hysteroscopy, then it is the omentum and indicates perforation. This diagnosis is to be ruled out before proceeding further. If the patient is under LA or spinal anesthesia, she may complain of sudden lower abdominal pain, nausea, irritability, or hemodynamic depression. For patients under GA, the anesthesiologist must concentrate on the video display of intrauterine cavity continuously and also be on the alert to pick up signs of uterine perforation. If uterine perforation is confirmed, a general surgeon may be called to assess the extent of damage to the uterus and/or urinary bladder and also the lower intestinal system.

2.2.3   Fluid Overload

The incidence of fluid overload during hysteroscopy ranges from 0.1% to 0.2% [17, 18], and fluid overload with consequent hyponatremia and hypoosmolality occurs in up to 6% of cases undergoing a surgical hysteroscopy procedure [21].

Typically, fluid overloading mimics the situation that the anesthesiologists encounter during transurethral resection of prostate (TURP) gland. However, there are few differences to consider; first, compared to the urinary bladder, the uterus is smaller in size, thick-walled, and relatively indistensible. Second, as opposed to TURP, saline irrigation is employed for non-operative hysteroscopy, and therefore, even with fluid overload, hyponatremia is seldom an issue. Third, higher irrigation pressures (80–150 mmHg) are required to distend the uterine cavity [3]. Fourth, because female steroids (estrogen) inhibit Na+/K+-ATP pump, premenopausal women are 25 times more likely to die or suffer from permanent brain damage following development of hyponatremic encephalopathy than their men undergoing transurethral resection of prostate (TURP) [22]. Therefore, hyponatremia management is to be critically considered each time irrigation solution without electrolytes is used for operative hysteroscopy. Interestingly, fluid overload has been reported even with use of low-volume irrigation fluid. There may be dysfunctional outflow irrigation channel that reduces fluid turnover. Also, there may be an opened up sinus which absorbs fluid rapidly under high distension pressure hysteroscopy. There are many ways that fluid overloading with distending fluid can be prevented (Table 2.4). The anesthesiologist should be geared up to treat fluid overload leading to congestive cardiac failure and pulmonary edema that ensues following large-volume hysteroscopy. The fluid overload treatment includes head-up position, dangling lower limbs, Lasix (40 mg), and morphine sulfate (15 mg). The hysteroscopy procedure must be abandoned at the earliest and the patient moved to intensive care for elective mechanical ventilation and continual management.

Table 2.4 Measures to avoid fluid overload	1. *Maintaining intrauterine distension pressure*
	– Gravity system of irrigation: Fluid hung 1–1.5 m above the uterus level
	– Distension pressure: 80–150, preferably, below resting mean blood pressure of patient
	– Controlling pressurized delivery system (pressure cuff around the fluid bag)
	– Monitoring and adjusting infusion pump pressure
	2. *Reducing systemic absorption of the distending fluid media*
	– Reducing volume of irrigation fluid
	– Administration of gonadotropin-releasing hormone (GnRH) analogues [23]
	– Injection of dilute vasopressin (8 mL 0.05 U/mL) into the cervix [24]
	3. *Advocating staged surgery if operative intervention is getting prolonged*
	4. *Use of intrauterine RF vaporization electrodes [25], intrauterine morcellator [26]*

2.2.4   Venous Air Embolism (VAE)

Since irrigation fluids and gases are administered with higher distension pressures to mitigate the impedance of a thick uterine wall, there is a possibility that sinuses may open up and gas/air can get into them [27, 28]. Therefore, it is extremely important to de-air the irrigation system lest the dead space air gets into systemic circulation through opened up sinuses. This situation, although rare, is a possibility during operative hysteroscopy involving fibromyoma excision. Therefore, a high degree of suspicion must be maintained to identify this early and to take emergent treatment actions. Further, the anesthesia technologist must be well-trained to avoid the situation where irrigation fluid bottle gets emptied without getting noticed. This is another potential source of VAE in patients undergoing hysteroscopy. In this regard to VAE diagnosis and effective management (central venous line insertion, patient positioning), endotracheal GA with end-tidal carbon dioxide monitoring is advantageous.

2.2.5   Deep Vein Thrombosis (DVT)

Due to the presence of a host of factors (estrogen, obesity, lithotomy position, use of anticoagulants to control bleeding during surgery) in females undergoing hysteroscopy procedure, DVT possibility cannot be ruled out. Therefore, proactive DVT prophylaxis is desirable. Preoperative application of mechanical insufflation device to the legs, keeping knees slightly flexed with padding under the knees, and pharmacologic cover (low molecular weight heparin administered the evening before) are keys to successful prevention of a DVT event [6].

2.3   Postanesthesia Recovery, Analgesia, and Hospital Discharge Management

It is imperative that use of short-acting and quick elimination anesthetic drugs would hasten emergence and recovery from anesthesia. However there are certain caveats to consider: first, women with a host of associated systemic illnesses and hormone therapy are more likely to suffer from postoperative nausea and vomiting (PONV). Therefore, a proactive approach to prevention and treatment of PONV is advisable, which may include preoperative pro-kinetics (per oral metoclopramide 10 mg and/or ranitidine 150 mg an hour before surgery) agents and antiemetic medications for the postoperative episode (intravenous dexamethasone 4 mg, ondansetron 4 mg). Second, the other potential problem after hysteroscopy is pain. Typically, the postoperative analgesia used for patients of hysteroscopy should be devoid of hangover, respiratory depression, or sedation [29]. In order to achieve a pain-free alert patient status, multimodal nonsteroidal analgesics (NSAIDs) (intravenous diclofenac 75 mg), paracetamol (intravenous, 1.0 g over 20 min), selective serotonin receptor uptake inhibitors (intravenous tramadol 100 mg), etc. In addition, the author administers microdose of midazolam (intravenous, 0.25 mg bolus) immediately following analgesic agent to minimize neuroplasticity that may trouble patients with pain when they reach home.

Over and above the responsive management to PONV and pain, close monitoring of patient's hemodynamics, oxygen saturation, respiration, level of consciousness, and ability to pass urine is required. Urine output monitoring is essential if large-volume irrigation is utilized and if patient has a pre-existing cardiac or respiratory ailment, is postmenopausal, or is on long-term hormone therapy. Early recovery lasting 6 h is crucial to the first phase of hospital discharge because only after that the patient may be relegated to step-down recovery. While the attendants can visit their patients here, the monitoring is continued. Of the several discharge criteria which are applied to assess patient's readiness for discharge, the postanesthesia discharge scoring system (PADSS score) applies for the post-hysteroscopy patients [30, 31]. In short, a patient who has passed urine, has taken oral liquids without any bloating/retching, is able to move around without orthostatic effects, and, most importantly, has an accompanying adult attendant can be safely discharged home.

Conclusions

Management of anesthesia for hysteroscopy remains an important responsibility for anesthesiologists. In order to maintain quality of overall care and secure safety of the patients during hysteroscopy procedure, the "absolute" (indication, positioning, irrigation fluid) and the "relative" (patient comorbidity, electrically energized equipment, complications) implications of anesthesia warrant sensitive and standardized management. The options for the type of anesthesia should be exercised in line with nature of intervention (elective, emergent), patient's choice, indication and intricacies of hysteroscopy, and the likelihood of emergent problems. To this effect, careful planning, immaculate conduct of anesthesia and hysteroscopy, the clarity of communication between anesthesiologist and the surgeon, and the postoperative care of the patient require consistent attention in detail.

References

1. Nagele F, Connor HO, Davies A, Badawy A, Mohamed H, Magos A. 2500 outpatient diagnostic hysteroscopies. Obstet Gynecol. 1996;88:87–92.
2. Hesla JS. Therapeutic hysteroscopy: indications and techniques. J Gynecol Surg. 2009;6:147.
3. Mushambi MC, Williamson K. Anaesthetic considerations for hysteroscopic surgery. Best Pract Res Clin Anaesthesiol. 2002;16:35–52.
4. Smith I, Kranke P, Murat I, Smith A, O'Sullivan G, Soriede E, et al. European society of Anesthesiology. Perioperative fasting in adults and children: guidelines from the European Society of Anaesthesiology. Eur J Anaesthesiol. 2011;28:556–69.
5. Murdoch JAC, Gan TJ. Anesthesia for hysteroscopy. Anesthesiol Clin North America. 2001;19:125–40.
6. Nelson G, Altman AD, Nick A, Meyer LA, Ramirez PT, Achtari C, et al. Guidelines for pre- and intraoperative care in gynecology/oncology surgery: enhanced recovery after surgery (ERAS) society recommendations - Part I. Gynecol Oncol. 2016;140:313–22.

7. Guida M, Pellicano M, Zullo F, Acunzo G, Lavitola G, Palomba S, et al. Outpatient hysteroscopy with bipolar electrode: a prospective, multicenter randomized study between local anaesthesia and conscious sedation. Hum Reprod. 2003;18:840–3.

8. Cooper NA, Khan KS, Clark TJ. Local anaesthesia for pain control during outpatient hysteroscopy: systematic review and meta-analysis. BMJ. 2010;340:c1130.

9. Florio P, Puzzutiello R, Filippeschi M, D'Onofrio P, Mereu L, Morelli R, et al. Low-dose spinal anesthesia with hyperbaric bupivacaine with intrathecal fentanyl for operative hysteroscopy: a case series study. J Minim Invasive Gynecol. 2012;19:107–12.

10. Jabbari A, Alijanpour E, Mir M, Bani Hashem N, Rabiea SM, Rupani MA. Post spinal puncture headache, an old problem and new concepts: review of articles about predisposing factors. Caspian J Intern Med. 2013;4:595–602.

11. Fleisch MC, Bremerich D, Schulte-Mattler W, Tannen A, Teichmann AT, Bader W, et al. The prevention of positioning injuries during gynecologic operations. Guideline of DGGG (S1-Level, AWMF Registry No. 015/077, February 2015). Geburtshilfe Frauenheilkd. 2015;75:792–807.

12. AAGL, et al. AAGL Practice Report: practice guidelines for the management of hysteroscopic distending media. J Minim Invasive Gynecol. 2013;20(2):137–48.

13. Pellicano M, Guida M, Zullo F, Lavitola G, Cirillo D, Nappi C. Carbon dioxide versus normal saline as a uterine distention medium for diagnostic vaginoscopic hysteroscopy in infertile patients: a prospective, randomized, multicenter study. Fertil Steril. 2003;79:418–21.

14. Mangar D. Anaesthetic implications of 32% dextran-70 (Hyskon) during hysteroscopy: hysteroscopy syndrome. Can J Anaesth. 1992;39:975–9.

15. Perlitz Y, Oettinger M, Karam K, Lipshitz B, Simon K. Anaphylactic shock during hysteroscopy using Hyskon solution: case report and review of adverse reactions and their treatment. Gynecol Obstet Invest. 1996;41:67–9.

16. Darwish AM, Hassan ZZ, Attia AM, Abdelraheem SS, Ahmed YM. Biological effects of distension media in bipolar versus monopolar resectoscopic myomectomy: a randomized trial. J Obstet Gynaecol Res. 2010;36:810–7.

17. Aydeniz B, Gruber IV, Schauf B, Kurek R, Meyer A, Wallwiener D. A multicenter survey of complications with 21,676 operative hysteroscopies. Eur J Obstet Gynecol Biol. 2002;104:160–4.

18. Jansen FW, Vredevoogd CB, van Ulzen K, Hermans J, Trimbos JB, Tribos-Kemper TC. Complications of hysteroscopy: a prospective, multicenter study. Obstet Gynecol. 2000;96:266–70.

19. Agostini A, Cravello L, Bretelle F, Shojai R, Roger V, Blanc B. Risk of uterine perforation during hysteroscopic surgery. J Am Assoc Gynecol Laparosc. 2002;9:264–7.

20. Mousa SA, Yassem AM, Alhadary HS, Sadek EES, Abdel-Hady EL-S. Hematological profile and transfusion requirement during hysteroscopic myomectomy: a comparative study between oxytocin and tranexamic acid infusion. Egypt J Anaesth. 2012;28:125–32.

21. Indman PD, Brooks PG, Cooper JM, Loffer FD, Valle RF, Vancaillie TG. Complications of fluid overload from resectoscopic surgery. J Am Assoc Gynaecol Laprosc. 1998;5:63–7.

22. Ayus JC, Wheeler JM, Arieff AI. Postoperative hyponatremic encephalopathy in menstruant women. Ann Intern Med. 1992;117:891–7.

23. Taskin O, Buhur A, Birincioglu M, et al. Endometrial N+, K+-ATPase pump function and vasopressin levels during hysteroscopic surgery in patients pre-treated with GnRH agonist. J Amm Assoc Gynecol Laparosc. 1998;5:119–24.

24. Corson SL, Brookes PG, Serden SP, Batzer FR, Gocial B. Effects of vasopressin administration during hysteroscopic surgery. J Reprod Med. 1994;39:419–23.

25. Vercellini P, Oldani S, Milesi M, Rossi M, Carinelli S, Crosignani PG. Endometrial ablation with a vaporizing electrode. Evaluation of in vivo effects. Acta Obstet Gynecol Scand. 1998;77:683–7.

26. Emanuel MH, Wamsteker K. The intrauterine morcellator: a new hysteroscopic operating technique to intrauterine polyps and myomas. J Minim Invasive Gynecol. 2005;12:62–6.

27. Stoloff DR, Isenberg RA, Brill AI. Venous air and gas emboli in operative hysteroscopy. J Am Assoc Gynecol Laprosc. 2001;8:181–92.
28. Corson SL, Brooks PG, Soderstrom RM. Gynecologic endoscopic gas embolism. Fertil Steril. 1996;65:529–33.
29. Mazzon I, Faviili A, Grasso M, Horvath S, Bini V, Renzo GCD. Pain in diagnostic hysteroscopy: a multivariate analysis after a randomized controlled trial. Fertil Steril. 2014;102:1398–403.
30. Trevisani L, Cifala V, Gilli G, Matarese V, Zelante A, Sartori S. Post-Anaesthetic Discharge Scoring System to assess patient recovery and discharge after colonoscopy. World J Gastrointest Endosc. 2013;5:502–7.
31. Pallumbo P, Tellan G, Perotti B, Pacille MA, Vietri F, Illuminati G. Modified PADSS (Post-Anaesthetic Discharge Scoring System) for monitoring outpatient discharge. Ann Ital Chir. 2013;84:661–5.

Indications and Contraindications of Hysteroscopy

3

Aanchal Agarwal

3.1 Introduction

Hysteroscopy literally means visualization of the cavity of the uterus using a camera. It is a very useful tool for a variety of problems presenting to a gynecologist/infertility specialist. It can be used both for diagnostic and curative purposes. However, diagnostic hysteroscopy alone is not logical and should be followed by corrective procedures in the same sitting wherever equipment as well as technical expertise is available. This saves time, cost, as well as exposure to repeated anesthesia. Hysteroscopic visualization is best in immediate post-menstrual period but can be performed in any phase of menstrual cycle (Fig. 3.1).

3.2 Diagnostic Hysteroscopy

It can be performed in two ways:

3.2.1 Conventional Inpatient Approach

Conventional inpatient approach, which is done under anesthesia, is also known as classic technique. It involves inserting a vaginal speculum to visualize the cervix, dilating the cervix with serial Hegar dilators, sounding the canal for uterocervical length, and then inserting the hysteroscope. Liquid distension medium such as normal saline is used to distend the cavity. This method requires general anesthesia since dilatation of the cervix is painful.

A. Agarwal, DGO, DNB, FNB (Rep Med)
Department of Infertility, IVF and Reproductive Medicine,
B L K Superspeciality Hospital, New Delhi, India

© Springer Nature Singapore Pte Ltd. 2018
S. Jain, D. B. Inamdar (eds.), *Manual of Fertility Enhancing Hysteroscopy*,
https://doi.org/10.1007/978-981-10-8028-9_3

Fig. 3.1 Panoramic view of uterine cavity on hysteroscopy showing the fundus and ostia

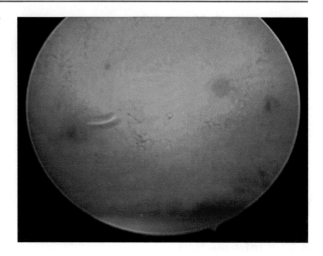

Table 3.1 The major differentiating features

	Conventional hysteroscopy	Office hysteroscopy	Operative hysteroscopy
Diameter of sheath	3.3–3.7 mm	<3 mm	8.7 mm
Speculum	Used	Not required	Used
Tenaculum	Used	Not required	Used
Cervical dilatation	Required	Not required	Required
Distension medium	Low-viscosity saline	Low-viscosity saline	High-viscosity glycine
Anesthesia	Required	Not required	Required

3.2.2 Modern Office Hysteroscopy

Modern office hysteroscopy also known as **vaginocervicohysteroscopy** or "no-touch" technique uses mini hysteroscopes. The "no-touch" method is preferable for office hysteroscopy since speculum and dilators are not used. Hysteroscope is introduced in the vaginal introitus, and a low-viscosity liquid distension medium (e.g., normal saline) is allowed to distend the vagina. This facilitates the direct visualization of external cervical os and with a narrow diameter scope; uterine cavity can be entered without cervical dilatation. This method of office hysteroscopy requires skill and technique and can be performed in majority of patients without any discomfort with a success rate of over 90%. However, presence of cervical stenosis is a contraindication to this procedure (Table 3.1).

Further advantage of office hysteroscopy is that the physical examination, transvaginal scan (TVS), and hysteroscopy can be combined in one outpatient sitting. Immediately after the hysteroscopy, a second TVS can be performed taking advantage of the intracavitary fluid for a contrast image of the uterus just like in a sonohysterosalpingogram.

3.3   Indications for Hysteroscopy (Table 3.2)

The major indications are described in detail as follows:

3.3.1   Space-Occupying Lesion (SOL) on Ultrasound or Filling Defect on Hysterosalpingography (HSG)

Such a shadow can be due to either an endometrial polyp or fibroid or intrauterine synechiae. Hysteroscopy remains the gold standard for diagnosis of such problems with an added advantage that correction can be done in the same sitting.

3.3.1.1 Endometrial Polyp

Polyps are seen as localized filling defect in the cavity on HSG and as SOL on ultrasound. Polyps can be functional or nonfunctional. They are also seen in patients receiving tamoxifen for breast cancer. On hysteroscopy, nonfunctional polyps are seen as white protuberances with branching fine vessels on the surface, whereas functional polyps are smaller and look similar to the surrounding endometrium. It has been found that hysteroscopic removal of polyps is far superior compared to blind curettage [1] as the latter can result in incomplete removal in many cases (Figs. 3.2 and 3.3).

Table 3.2 Indications of diagnostic and operative hysteroscopy

Indications of diagnostic hysteroscopy	Indications of operative hysteroscopy
Gynecological indications	1. Polypectomy
1. SOL (space-occupying lesion) on pelvic ultrasound or filling defect on hysterosalpingography	2. Myomectomy
	3. Adhesiolysis
	4. Resection of uterine septum/ metroplasty
2. Abnormal uterine bleeding	5. Endometrial ablation/resection
3. Endometrial hyperplasia and malignancy	6. Cannulation of the fallopian tubes
4. Endometrial atrophy	7. Falloposcopy
5. Endometrial tuberculosis	8. Removal of a lost IUCD
6. Recurrent miscarriage	9. Site-specific endometrial injury before IVF/ET
7. Congenital uterine anomaly	10. Treatment of cervical and interstitial pregnancy
8. Asherman's syndrome	
9. Post-adhesiolysis check hysteroscopy	11. Treatment of missed abortion/ retained products of conception
10. Follow-up of medical or surgical treatment	
11. Lost intrauterine contraceptive device (IUCD)	12. Tubal sterilization
Indications specific to infertility	13. Improving fertility of hydrosalpinx by blocking cornual end
12. Unexplained infertility	
13. Pre-assisted reproductive techniques (pre-ART)	14. Hysteroscopy-assisted embryo transfer (SEED/HEED)
14. Along with diagnostic laparoscopy for complete evaluation of the pelvis	
15. Embryo evaluation (embryoscopy)	

Fig. 3.2 Hysteroscopy
picture of a fleshy polyp

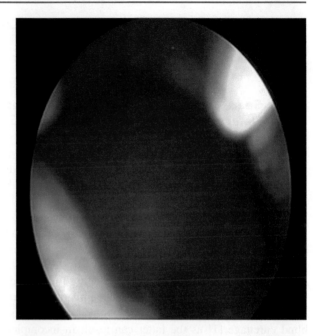

Fig. 3.3 A sessile polyp on
hysteroscopy

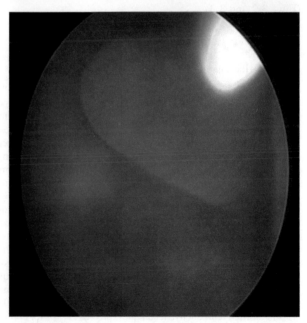

This is further substantiated by the review of literature by Salim et al. according
to which hysteroscopic resection is the most effective management for endometrial
polyps and allows histologic assessment, whereas blind biopsy or curettage has low
diagnostic accuracy and should not be performed [2].

3.3.1.2 Myoma

Fibroid or myoma uterus can be classified in various ways:

1. Sessile or pedunculated as per the absence or presence of stalk
2. According to the location with respect to cavity, they can be classified as Type 0 (T0), Type 1 (T1), and Type 2 (T2) as per the European Society of Gynecological Endoscopy classification

Type 0 myomas are entirely within the uterine cavity and appear as white spherical masses with a network of thin fragile vessels on surface. These can be dealt with easily using a hysteroscopic scissors/resectoscope.

Type 1 myomas are more than 50% in the cavity and partially embedded in the myometrium. The intracavitary part can be removed using loop on resectoscope or a hysteroscopic morcellator. For deep-seated big myomas requiring extensive resection, laparoscopic/USG guidance should be taken. Complete resection might require more than one procedure in large myomas. Nd:YAG (neodymium:yttrium aluminum garnet) laser/radiofrequency electrodesiccation may be needed for destroying the remaining portion of myoma.

Type 2 myomas are deep-seated with <50% component in the cavity. These are best removed through laparoscopy or laparotomy.

Best results are seen in myomas which are 5 cm or less in diameter and entirely intracavitary (Type 0) (Figs. 3.4, 3.5, and 3.6).

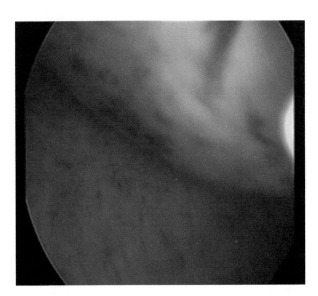

Fig. 3.4 Submucous fibroid on hysteroscopy

Fig. 3.5 Slicing of fibroid
using resectoscope and
loop

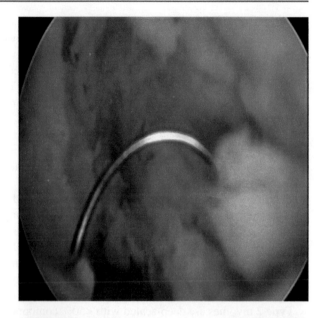

Fig. 3.6 Removal of
myoma in fragments

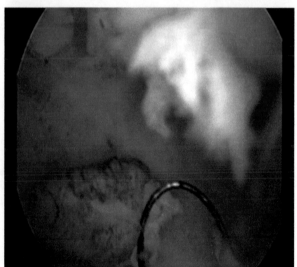

3.3.2 Intrauterine Synechiae

Intrauterine Synechiae are bands of adhesions between anterior and posterior
wall of the uterus. Most common causes are trauma or infection such as tuberculosis (TB) or an estrogen-deprived environment as in abortion/PPH [3]. The
risk is as high as one in five women after abortion [4]. Tuberculosis affecting
endometrium also leads to varying degree of synechiae obliterating the uterine

cavity. These are visible on HSG as filling defects which may vary from minimal to severe and obliterate the endometrial cavity partially or completely (Figs. 3.7 and 3.8).

Fig. 3.7 Thick band of intrauterine synechiae on hysteroscopy

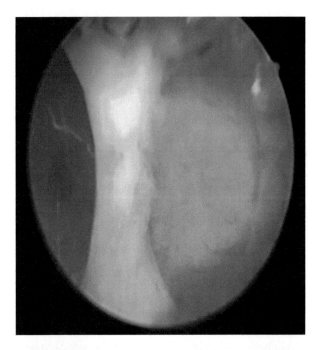

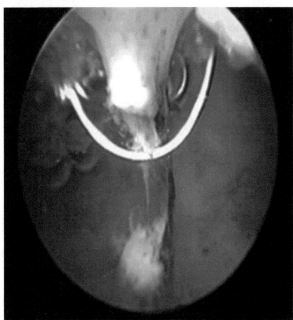

Fig. 3.8 Resection of synechia using loop

Hysteroscopic resection of thick synechiae is a technically challenging surgery because multiple vascular channels are opened up on cutting the band. This further increases the chances of intravascular absorption of distending medium which in case of glycine can lead to life-threatening complications. Complete removal of extensive adhesions may require repeated procedures. Sometimes check hysteroscopy is needed after an adhesiolysis procedure. Baruah and associates studied reproductive outcome following hysteroscopic adhesiolysis in patients with infertility due to Asherman's syndrome and found a conception rate of 44.3% and a live birthrate of 86.1% [5]. However, there was no conception in patients who needed repeat adhesiolysis.

3.4   Abnormal Uterine Bleeding (AUB)

AUB encompasses a variety of menstrual problems which can manifest in different forms. Hysteroscopy is indicated in the following situations:

- Excessive amount or duration of bleeding, commonly in women of age 40 years or more
- Excessive bleeding not responsive to medical therapy even in women of age <40 years
- Intermenstrual bleeding with a normal cervical smear
- Postcoital bleeding with a normal cervical smear
- Postmenopausal bleeding or endometrial thickness of ≥4 mm in a postmenopausal lady
- Oligomenorrhea or amenorrhea in reproductive age group

In all these situations, hysteroscopy helps in making a diagnosis as well as in taking a targeted biopsy from a suspicious area. In cases of thick endometrium where malignancy has been ruled out, hysteroscopic endometrial resection (TCRE) can cure the problem thus avoiding a potential hysterectomy. This procedure is not suitable for women desiring fertility in the future.

However, for a woman in reproductive age group, oligomenorrhea or amenorrhea is usually due to intrauterine synechiae or atrophic endometrium. These can be diagnosed as well as cured with hysteroscopy.

3.5   Congenital Uterine Anomalies

The commonest uterine anomalies encountered in clinical practice are complete or partial uterine septum, bicornuate uterus, uterus didelphys, and transverse vaginal septum. Most of them can be picked up on an HSG. Sometimes it is difficult to differentiate a septum from a bicornuate uterus on imaging. Though MRI has a high accuracy, laparo-hysteroscopy is the gold standard. On laparoscopy, a septate uterus has a broad fundus, whereas a bicornuate uterus is heart shaped. These anomalies can cause recurrent pregnancy loss or preterm labor, whereas a transverse vaginal septum can cause infertility. Resection of uterine septum can be done hysteroscopically. The technique

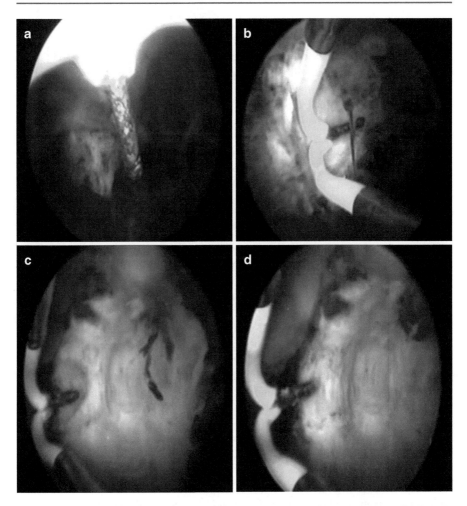

Fig. 3.9 (**a–d**) Hysteroscopic resection of the septum from one end to the other using Collin's knife

was first described by Decherney and associates in 1986 [6] and then by March and Israel in 1987 [7]. It can be done using scissors/resectoscope/Nd:YAG laser. The septum is cut from below and upward. It is best to do it under laparoscopic guidance. It is always better to undercorrect a septum rather than overdo and perforate (Fig. 3.9).

3.6   Hysteroscopy in Infertility

Unexplained infertility can be due to thin synechiae in the uterine cavity which may not be visible on ultrasound/HSG. Other causes could be endometritis or atrophic endometrium. Endometritis can only be picked up on direct visualization during a hysteroscopy; ultrasound is not useful in this condition. Strawberry hue with branching vasculature is typical of endometritis.

Quite a lot of clinicians consider hysteroscopy mandatory before an IVF cycle due to the abovementioned reasons. First of all, it helps in obtaining direct view of the uterine cavity starting from the cervical canal to the uterine fundus and diagnosing small focal or expanded lesions otherwise missed on imaging. Secondly, it gives useful information about the route to follow during embryo transfer thus avoiding a traumatic transfer.

As per the analysis of 2500 office-based diagnostic hysteroscopies before IVF by Karayalcin et al., 77.1% patients had a normal uterine cavity, while the remainder of 22.9% demonstrated endometrial pathology on hysteroscopy. Of the patients with endometrial pathology, 7.68% patients had endometrial polyps, 3.84% patients had submucosal fibroids, 1.24% had polypoid endometria, 1.08% patients had intra-uterine adhesions, and 2.92% patients had uterine septa. These results were seen in unselected population, and a significant percentage of patients had evidence of uterine pathology that may have impaired the success of IVF [8]. Endometrial scratching, with or without hysteroscopy, has been documented to improve implantation in previous failed IVF cycles [9, 10].

In tubal factor infertility, the lumen of the fallopian tubes can be evaluated through hysteroscopic **falloposcopy** where a narrow lumen scope is introduced through the cornual end and mucosal folds inside tubal lumina are directly visualized. This can help in prognosticating regarding possibility of a spontaneous pregnancy.

For **embryoscopy**, rigid mini endoscopes can now be introduced transabdominally and trans-uterinally to observe the embryo in situ with better resolution. As the technology advances, the possibility of a practical transcervical method for embryoscopy remains on the horizon. As mini endoscopes become accepted for intrauterine visualization, the transfer of gametes, zygotes, or embryos under visual control may become a reality.

3.7   Recurrent Pregnancy Loss (RPL)

RPL may be caused by anatomic abnormalities of the cervix or uterine cavity. These may be either congenital or acquired. Congenital causes include mullerian duct fusion abnormalities, the commonest of which are incomplete uterine septum and abnormalities caused by in utero DES exposure. Acquired anatomic abnormalities include intrauterine adhesions, myoma, and endometritis. These may not be picked up on ultrasound or HSG many times. First trimester losses in these conditions are mainly due to abnormal placentation. The endometrium overlying these lesions is poorly developed which leads to poor vascularization of the placenta. Hysteroscopic correction has shown to improve pregnancy outcome in the abovementioned conditions [11, 12].

3.8   Cannulation of the Fallopian Tubes

Cannulation of the fallopian tubes under hysteroscopic guidance is done for treating interstitial obstruction due to mucus plug or debris or spasm. This procedure is combined with laparoscopy. A Teflon cannula with a metal obturator is introduced through operating channel of the hysteroscopic sheath and gently advanced through the tubal ostia till resistance is encountered or till cornua is reached. The obturator is then withdrawn and dye is injected through the catheter. Mucus plug or debris or thin adhesions get dislodged by pressure, and the flow of dye through the fimbrial end can be seen simultaneously through the laparoscope.

3.9 Hysteroscopic Tubal Sterilization

This method of permanent sterilization uses a micro insert consisting of soft stainless steel inner coil and a dynamic nickel-titanium alloy outer coil known as Essure. The device is introduced into the uterus with a 5 mm operating channel hysteroscope and guided into the proximal section of the fallopian tube at the uterotubal junction. Fibrous tissue grows into it with time occluding the tubes permanently.

3.10 Treatment of Missed Abortion/Retained Products of Conception

When an early first trimester pregnancy termination fails and histological examination of the products of conception does not demonstrate chorionic villi, an ectopic pregnancy should be suspected, particularly if the pregnancy test is persistently positive. In such a case, when laparoscopy fails to demonstrate tubal/ovarian/peritoneal pathology consistent with an ectopic pregnancy, hysteroscopy may be of value.

The reason may be early gestation in an anomalous uterus, such as a septate uterus with an early pregnancy at a site that was not curetted. Hysteroscopy can guide selective suction aspiration for termination of the missed pregnancy. This approach has been greatly facilitated with the use of concomitant sonography.

3.11 Removal of Impacted or Lost IUCD

Sometimes the thread of an IUCD is not visible in the vagina. Such a lost IUCD or an impacted foreign body can be removed using a specially designed hook or a toothed curette under hysteroscopic guidance.

3.12 Contraindications of Hysteroscopy

Absolute	Relative
1. Intrauterine pregnancy	1. Inexperienced surgeon
2. Advanced genital tract cancer because of a risk of dissemination of cancer cells. However, it may be used for diagnosis and management in early stage	2. Heavy uterine bleeding
	3. Cardiovascular disease
	4. Contraindications to anesthesia (for routine/operative hysteroscopy)
3. Active pelvic infection	
4. Cervical atresia	
5. Recent perforation	

3.13   Absolute Contraindications

Absolute contraindications for hysteroscopy are those where this procedure should not be performed at all. If it is performed, there is a very high risk to the patient. These include the presence of an intrauterine pregnancy which has a very high possibility of getting the fetus misplaced and getting aborted. In cases of an active genital infection and cancer, the disease can get disseminated. Since the flow of fluid distension medium is from the uterine cavity through the fallopian tubes into peritoneal cavity, it can carry the infectious microorganism/cancerous cells along with leading to dissemination.

3.14   Relative Contraindications

Relative contraindications for infertility are those where the procedure may cause harm or may be inconclusive. In cases of heavy uterine bleeding, it may not be possible to see anything at all except blood, and the procedure becomes inconclusive. Similarly, an inexperienced surgeon may not be able to maneuver the equipment properly and may cause a perforation. In case of cardiovascular disease, fluid overload, more so high viscosity fluid during operative procedure, can become life threatening. One has to keep a careful record of fluid input, output, and fluid balance.

Conclusion

Hysteroscopy is indicated in any situation in which an intrauterine pathology is suspected. It provides direct visualization of the uterine cavity and remains the gold standard for diagnosis and treatment of these lesions. Since it can be performed in office, it may be offered as a first-line diagnostic tool for evaluation of uterine cavity in patients with abnormal uterine bleeding and infertility. As an office procedure, the combination of TVS, hysteroscopy, and contrast sonography is the most powerful screening tool for detecting intracavitary abnormalities.

References

1. Gebauer G, Hafnee A, Siebzehnrubl E, et al. Role of hysteroscopy in detection & extraction of endometrial polyps: results of a prospective study. Am J Obstet Gynecol. 2002;186:1104.
2. Salim S, Won H, Nesbitt-Hawes E, Campbell N, Abbott J. Diagnosis and management of endometrial polyps: a critical review of literature. J Minim Invasive Gynecol. 2011;18(5):569–81.
3. Schenker JG. Etiology of and therapeutic approach to synechia uteri. Eur J Obstet Gynecol Reprod Biol. 1996;65(1):109.
4. Hooker AB, Lemmers M, Thurkow AL, Heymans MW, Opmeer BC, Brölmann HA, et al. Systematic review and meta-analysis of intrauterine adhesions after miscarriage: prevalence, risk factors and long-term reproductive outcome. Hum Reprod Update. 2014;20(2):262.

5. Roy KK, Baruah J, Sharma JB, Kumar S, Kachawa G, Singh N. Reproductive outcome following hysteroscopic adhesiolysis in patients with infertility due to Asherman's syndrome. Arch Gynecol Obstet. 2010;281(2):355–61.
6. Decherney AH, Russell JB, Graebe RA. etal. Resectoscopic management of mullerian fusion defects. Fertil Steril. 1986;45:7.
7. March CM, Israel R. Hysteroscopic management of recurrent abortion caused by septate uterus. Am J Obstet Gynecol. 1987;156:834.
8. Karayalcin R, Ozcan S, Moraloglu O, Ozyer S, Mollamahmutoglu L, etal BS. Results of 2500 office-based diagnostic hysteroscopies before IVF. Reprod Biomed Online. 2010;20(5):689–93.
9. Simon C, et al. 'The Scratching case': systematic reviews and meta-analyses, the back door for evidence based medicine. Hum Reprod. 2014;29:1618–21.
10. Nastri CO, Lensen SF, Gibreel A, Raine-Fenning N, Ferriani RA, Bhattacharya S, Martins WP. Endometrial injury in women undergoing assisted reproductive techniques. Cochrane Database Syst Rev. 2015;(3):CD009517. https://doi.org/10.1002/14651858.CD009517.pub3.
11. Propst AM, Hill JA III. Anatomic factors associated with RPL. Semin Reprod Med. 2000;18:341–50.
12. Homer HA, Li T-C, Cooke ID. The septate uterus: a review of management and reproductive outcome. Fertil Steril. 2000;73:1–14.

Hysteroscopy and Fertility

4

Nameeta Mokashi Bhalerao

4.1 Introduction

In recent years, endoscopic techniques have gained much momentum in all branches of the medical field for the diagnosis and treatment of diseases. The main benefit is the minimally invasive surgical course of diagnosis and simultaneous therapeutic relief apart from direct optical judgment of body cavities. In gynecology too, although laparoscopy has been very well established now, hysteroscopy unfortunately still has been struggling to get accepted as a routine maneuver.

Though over the years hysteroscopy has proved itself to be highly useful for the evaluation and management of intrauterine diseases, its position in current fertility practice continues to be a matter of much debate.

In this chapter of "Hysteroscopy and Fertility," we will be having a general overview on the role that hysteroscopy can portray in the practice of fertility.

Infertility is "a disease of the reproductive system defined by the failure to achieve a clinical pregnancy after 12 months or more of regular unprotected sexual intercourse" according to the International Committee for Monitoring Assisted Reproductive Technology (ICMART) and the World Health Organization (WHO) [1].

In general, investigations are conducted after 12 months of exposure. However, some cases including those with oligomenorrhea, history of pelvic surgery, tubal infection, or chemotherapy require earlier investigations. For women older than 35 years, investigations should be started after 6 months of attempts [2].

Each member of the couple should undergo basic infertility investigations including assessment of the uterine cavity, fallopian tubes, ovarian function and reserve, and semen analysis. Among the various treatment options of ovulation induction, timed intercourse, intrauterine insemination, and in vitro fertilization, the latter is proving to widely represent the treatment choice for several conditions like

N. M. Bhalerao, MBBS, MS (ObGy), DNB, FNB, PGDMLE
Nova IVI Fertility Services, Pune, Maharashtra, India

© Springer Nature Singapore Pte Ltd. 2018
S. Jain, D. B. Inamdar (eds.), *Manual of Fertility Enhancing Hysteroscopy*,
https://doi.org/10.1007/978-981-10-8028-9_4

unexplained infertility, male factor, endometriosis, and ovarian dysfunction resistant to ovulation induction apart from the undisputed tubal infertility cases [3].

The introduction of in vitro fertilization (IVF), one of the major medical breakthroughs of the twentieth century, has over the years proved to be a viable treatment option for several forms of infertility. Since the first successful live birth through IVF in 1978, the use of IVF and its success rate too have steadily increased resulting in around five million children born utilizing the technology [4]. Although the IVF success rate has seen an improvement over the preceding years, majority of the cycles still fail in giving a live birth; only 25–30% of cycles of IVF and intracytoplasmic sperm injection (ICSI) lead to a live birth [5]. Despite continuing medical improvements and advancements, there persist the challenges of unexplained or repeated implantation failures [6].

4.2   In Search of the Missing Link

Notwithstanding the huge investment in research and developments of the technologies involved in assisted reproduction, infertility specialists continue to face challenges of maximizing the implantation rates [7, 8].

Toward these untiring attempts, it is crucial to remember that a satisfactory exploration of the uterine cavity is a necessary and basic step in infertility work-up given that:

1. The uterine cavity and moreover the endometrium are fundamental for the embryo implantation and normal placentation [1, 9].
2. Intrauterine lesions are prevalent in almost 40–50% of infertile women which is proven to compromise spontaneous fertility and pregnancy rate in ART [8].

Currently, tools to assess the uterine cavity include transvaginal ultrasound (TVS), gel or saline infusion sonography (GIS or SIS), hysterosalpingography (HSG), and hysteroscopy.

Among these, the gold standard technique for uterine factor evaluation is hysteroscopy, as it facilitates not only a direct visualization of the uterine cavity but also a faultless detection of various pathological disorders and the treatment of any detected abnormality. This is unlike the other indirect and purely diagnostic techniques of TVS, SIS/GIS, and HSG [1, 10].

4.2.1   Hysteroscopy vs. TVS and HSG

TVS and HSG have been proposed to be the primary diagnostic tools for uterine cavity abnormalities, but many studies have clearly demonstrated several drawbacks with their efficacy.

4.2.1.1 Hysteroscopy vs. TVS

Transvaginal 2D and 3D ultrasounds are the primary [1] screening tool for uterine evaluation and have a valuable role for diagnosis of myometrial disorders and

Mullerian anomalies. But with normal ultrasound findings too, pathological intra-cavitary lesions affecting reproduction may be missed and then get detected at hysteroscopy [11, 12].

1. In comparison with hysteroscopy, bidimensional (2D) ultrasonography (USG) is said to have 84.5% sensitivity, 98.7% specificity, 98% positive predictive value, and 89.2% negative predictive value [1, 13].
2. Machine and operator variables may miss diagnosing submucosal fibroids especially in the presence of multiple fibroids or may be less specific in differentiating a polyp from hyperplastic overgrown endometrium [1]
3. Bidimensional USG may also not differentiate between congenital uterine malformations [1, 14].

4.2.1.2 Hysteroscopy vs. HSG

1. HSG suffers from a lower sensitivity and specificity in comparison with hysteroscopy.
2. HSG appearances may vary depending on the phase of the menstrual cycle or growth status of the endometrium. Air bubbles, mucus, and menstrual debris may pose as artifacts or filling defects, hence giving false-positive results, or an excess contrast media injected may obliterate shadows of small endometrial lesions giving false-negative results.
3. Studies have shown a coherence of only about 65% between findings diagnosed with HSG and hysteroscopy [15]. Almost 1/3 of the patients interpreted as normal through HSG are detected to have a uterine abnormality through diagnostic hysteroscopy, so HSG might miss significant factors affecting reproductive performance or sometimes may overdiagnose not so significant factors [16, 17] (Table 4.1).

With the low accuracy rates of other diagnostic modalities, hysteroscopy definitely deserves the upper hand for confidently detecting any possible intrauterine pathology.

Overall, comparative studies of TVS or HSG showed unacceptably high false-negative rates, low positive predictive values, and poor diagnostic accuracy values in the evaluation of uterine cavity abnormalities. False-negative or normal HSG/USG may lead to false reassurance and result in lower than expected conception rate [1].

4.2.2 The Delayed Evolution of Hysteroscopy

Although hysteroscopy is widely considered to be the gold standard for the uterine cavity evaluation, worldwide it continues to be considered a second-line procedure for the uterine factor in infertile women (NICE, [22]), this being mainly related to its invasiveness and cost [23] as compared to TVS [1].

It has been a long and difficult way for hysteroscopy to gain acceptance [24] because of:

Table 4.1 Diagnostic capabilities of various tools evaluating uterine cavity

All units (in %)	2D USG	3D USG	2D USG polyp	3D polyp <5 mm	3D polyp >5 mm	HSG	HSG	Hysteroscopy Polyp	Hysteroscopy Fibroid
Diagnostic accuracy		84.1		45.5	85.7			97.6	100
Sensitivity	84.5	68.2	19–96	91.5	91.5	75.2	97	100	100
Specificity	98.7	91.5	53–100	82.8	90.7	41.4	23	96.8	100
PPV	98	79	75–100	55.6	60		44		
NPV	89	86	87–97	87.8	97.7		10		
References	[1, 13]	[14]	[18]	[14]	[14]	[19]	[20]	[14, 21]	[14, 21]

- Organ-specific problems
  1. Uterine cavity is a virtual cavity.
  2. The endometrium is very fragile.
  3. Resorption (vascular, peritoneal) and loss (cervix, tubes) of distension medium.
- Technique-specific problems
  1. Instrument: diameter and optical quality (image diameter, brightness, angle of view, field of view, resolution)
  2. Distension medium
  3. Video documentation
  4. Slow learning curve

Given the multiple advantages of hysteroscopy in improving the uterine factor contribution to successful implantation, it is time we take up hysteroscopy more frequently.

4.3   Indications of Hysteroscopy in Infertility [25]

1. Diagnostic
   (a) Abnormal uterine bleeding
   (b) Suspicious intrauterine lesions diagnosed on ultrasound/filling defects on HSG
   (c) Recurrent implantation failure
2. Therapeutic
   (a) Endocervical and/or endometrial polyps
   (b) Submucous and some intramural fibroids
   (c) Intrauterine adhesions
   (d) Mullerian anomalies (uterine septum)
   (e) Retained intrauterine devices/foreign body/products of conception

4.4   Contraindications to Hysteroscopy [25]

1. Viable intrauterine pregnancy
2. Active pelvic infection (including genital herpes infection)
3. Diagnosed cases of cervical or uterine cancer

4.5   Procedure of Hysteroscopy

4.5.1   Prior Work-Up

Before hysteroscopy, the standard investigations including Pap smear, vaginal bacteriologic tests, hemogram, and blood sugar level are done [25].

Routine antibiotic prophylaxis is not recommended for hysteroscopy as the risk of post hysteroscopy infection is <1% [22].

4.5.2   Procedure [24]

Patient is given a lithotomy position. Under all aseptic and sterile precautions, correct alignment of instruments is confirmed by free flow of distension medium. Hysteroscope is introduced intracervically channeling its path from the external cervical os and under visual guidance through the cervical canal across the internal cervical os. The passage through the cervical channel generally is the trickiest part of the total examination. On passage through the internal os, a resistance frequently has to be overcome before the uterine cavity is reached. By slowly turning the instrument along its axis, the tubal ostia can be clearly visualized with the 12° or 30° optic. Noting the state of the endometrium, its vascularity, the adequacy of the cavity, free flow of medium across the bilateral ostia, and any abnormalities is done along with complete documentation. The cervical canal is mainly inspected while withdrawing the instrument. The entire examination usually is accomplished within a few minutes.

4.5.3   Images of Normal and Pathological Uterine Cavities Diagnosed on Hysteroscopy (Figs. 4.1, 4.2, 4.3, 4.4, 4.5, and 4.6)

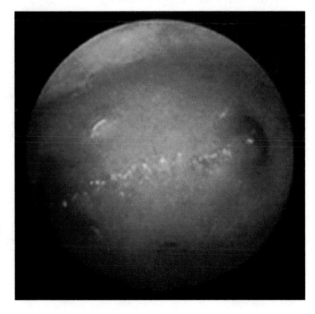

Fig. 4.1 Normal uterine cavity. Source: "Office mini-hysteroscopy," by Campo R et al. 1999, Human Reproduction Update; 5(1):73–81. Copyright 1999. Reproduced with permission from Oxford University Press

Fig. 4.2 Hypervascularization often seen in intrauterine myoma. Source: "Office mini-hysteroscopy," by Campo R et al. 1999, Human Reproduction Update; 5(1):73–81. Copyright 1999. Reproduced with permission from Oxford University Press

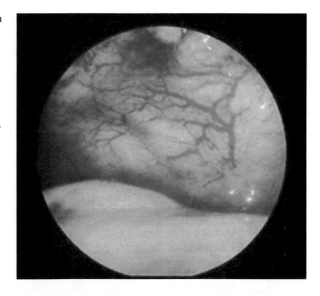

Fig. 4.3 Strawberry appearance. Source: "Office mini-hysteroscopy," by Campo R et al. 1999, Human Reproduction Update; 5(1):73–81. Copyright 1999. Reproduced with permission from Oxford University Press

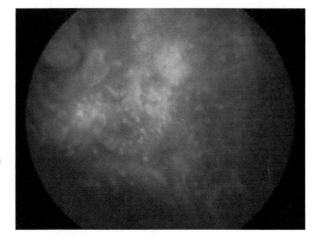

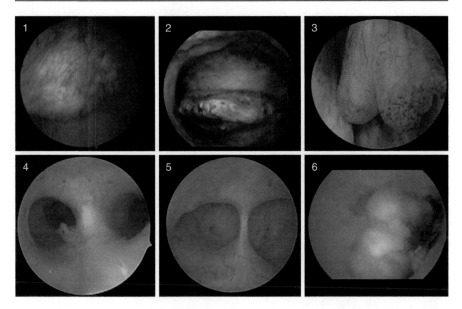

Fig. 4.4 Major pathologies: (1) submucous myoma, (2, 3) endometrial polyp, (4) uterine septum, (5) intrauterine adhesions, (6) placental remnants. Source "Implementation of hysteroscopy in an infertility clinic: The one-stop uterine diagnosis and treatment" by Campo R et al. 2014, Facts Views Vis Obgyn; 6(4): 235–239. Copyright 2014. Reproduced with permission from R Campo

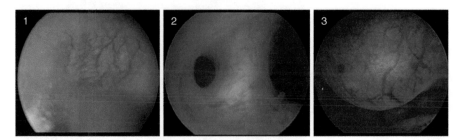

Fig. 4.5 Subtle lesions. (1) Focal hypervascularization, (2) cavity deformation, (3) mucosal elevation. Source "Implementation of hysteroscopy in an infertility clinic: The one-stop uterine diagnosis and treatment" by Campo R et al. 2014, Facts Views Vis Obgyn; 6(4): 235–239. Copyright 2014. Reproduced with permission from R Campo

Fig. 4.6 Hysteroscopy findings in adenomyosis: superficial openings within cavity and endometrial hypervascularization. Source: "Office Hysteroscopy and Adenomyosis" by Molinas CR 2006 [26]. Best Practice and Research Clinical Obstetrics and Gynecology; 20:557–567. Copyright 2006. Reproduced with permission from Elsevier

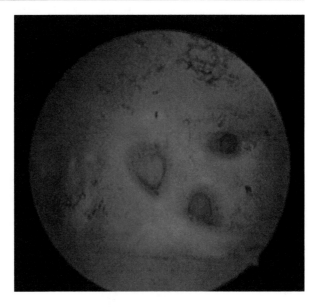

4.6 Mechanisms of Fertility-Enhancing Effects of Hysteroscopy

1. It permits reliable objective visual assessment of the cervical canal and uterine cavity apart from providing the opportunity to correct any abnormality found in the same setting. Most commonly encountered intrauterine pathologies are adhesions, endometrial polyps, submucous fibroids, endometritis, and uterine malformations [1, 6, 27] (Fig. 4.7).
   - Facilitates future embryo transfers: Embryo transfer is a very crucial step of IVF, and evidence outlays that the technical ease of this procedure has a big impact on avoiding eliciting uterine contractions and hence undue embryo expulsion. Hysteroscopy evaluates the direction/course/morphology of the cervical canal and uterine cavity so that due planning and maneuvering can be undertaken to lessen the tediousness or enhance the smoothness of embryo transfers [28].
   - Contemporaneous lysis of cervical adhesions [1].
   - The inevitable endometrial injury caused during uterine instrumentation invokes a post-traumatic reaction releasing cytokines and growth factors apart from modulating the expression of genes facilitating implantation like glycodelin-A, laminin, integrins, and matrix metalloproteinase [1].
   - Activates pro-implantation factors like leukocytes, cytokines, chemokines and other unknown endometrial factors [29, 30].
   - Pressure dilatation of the uterine cavity and tubes is also said to be effective in improving fertility [31].

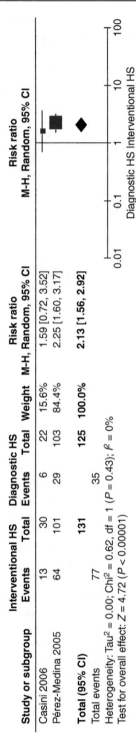

Study or subgroup	Interventional HS		Diagnostic HS		Weight	Risk ratio M-H, Random, 95% CI	Risk ratio M-H, Random, 95% CI
	Events	Total	Events	Total			
Casini 2006	13	30	6	22	15.6%	1.59 [0.72, 3.52]	
Pérez-Medina 2005	64	101	29	103	84.4%	2.25 [1.60, 3.17]	
Total (95% CI)		**131**		**125**	**100.0%**	**2.13 [1.56, 2.92]**	
Total events	77		35				

Heterogeneity: Tau^2 = 0.00; Chi^2 = 0.62, df = 1 (P = 0.43); I^2 = 0%
Test for overall effect: Z = 4.72 (P < 0.00001)

Diagnostic HS   Interventional HS

Infertile women affected by uterine fibroids or endometrial polyps. Operative versus diagnostic hysteroscopy. Pregnancy rate.

Fig. 4.7 Forest plot depicting benefit of hysteroscopy in increasing pregnancy rates after polypectomy or myomectomy. Source: "Efficacy of hysteroscopy in improving reproductive outcomes of infertile couples: a systematic review and meta-analysis" by Sardo Atillo et al. 2016. Human Reproduction Update; 22:479–496. Copyright 2016. Reproduced with permission from Oxford University Press

2. Saline Irrigation of the cavity may also have a beneficial effect. This may help to mechanically remove harmful anti-adhesive glycoprotein molecules on the endometrial surface involved in endometrial receptivity [i.e., cyclooxygenase-2 (COX-2), mucin-1 (MUC-1), and integrin aVb3] [1].

4.7   Conventional vs. Outpatient Hysteroscopy [24]

For a broad universal implementation, it is crucial to organize the hysteroscopic evaluation with a similar technical ease as with transvaginal ultrasound and with comparable patient compliance. One-stop uterine diagnosis approach has a potential to become technically facilitative diagnostic and therapeutic tool for both patients and clinicians. Minimizing the potential drawbacks is even more crucial. Hence, the concept of office hysteroscopy is becoming popular and preferred by both doctors and patients alike (Table 4.2).

The one-stop see-and-treat approach opens an attractive advanced dimension to the screening, diagnosis, and treatment of uterine pathology in the infertile patient.

Moreover, the new technical developments (atraumatic insertion, video camera, high-resolution small-diameter mini hysteroscopes, photo documentation, distension medium) raise the chance that hysteroscopy, both diagnostic and operative, may become established as a routine procedure by every gynecologist. The new generation of mini endoscopes, both rigid and microfiber systems, has excellent to acceptable optical qualities with a large image diameter, sufficient brightness, good resolution, and a field of view which allows panoramic sight [24].

With increasing experience and widespread use of outpatient hysteroscopy, a variety of intrauterine pathologies are now amenable to outpatient treatment, like polyp excision, submucous fibroid myomectomy, and adhesion excision. Outpatient services result in substantial benefits to patients, their employers, and society. These relate to time off home and work, travel and childcare arrangements, and cost savings to the healthcare service [32].

Table 4.2 Comparison between conventional and outpatient or office hysteroscopy [24]

	Conventional hysteroscopy	Outpatient/office hysteroscopy
Anesthesia/analgesia	General anesthesia	Not required
Instrument diameter	5 mm	2.9 mm
Cervical dilatation, speculum, tenaculum	Required	Atraumatic vagino-cervico insertion (no touch) Hence, not required
Patient compliance	Good	Better
		One-stop, see-and-treat technique

4.8   Potential of Hysteroscopy in Infertility

As having highlighted before, the evaluation of the uterine capacity for reproduction is an imperative step during infertility work-up, either during initial assessment or when any ART procedure is scheduled. In fact, intrauterine lesions are more common in infertile women (around 50%) [8, 33], compromising spontaneous conceptions as well as reducing success rates in assisted reproduction. So, a screening procedure can definitely be taken as useful.

The reliable visual assessment of the cervical canal and uterine cavity and the opportunity to perform corrective therapy in the same setting are favorable in enhancing success rates. Moreover, many investigators suggest routine pre-IVF hysteroscopy to ensure normalcy of the uterine cavity before embryo transfer to enhance success rates of ART [16, 34, 35] (Fig. 4.8).

Nevertheless, the routine use of the infertility work-up is still under debate. The RCOG [36], ESHRE (2000) [37], and NICE [22] guidelines do not recommend hysteroscopy as an initial screening investigation in infertility unless clinically indicated and have stated it as a grade B recommendation (RCOG 2004) [38].

In contrast to this, the current evidence is giving an increasing attention to the "time to pregnancy," already defined as "an essential conception of human reproduction." The prolonged time to pregnancy is becoming a crucial issue in the infertility work-up due to the dramatic increase in the mean age of women who attempt spontaneous conception and ART treatments. This social phenomenon has to be given consideration in light of the relevant acceleration of ovarian aging as well as the increase in the aneuploidy rates above 35 years of age [1].

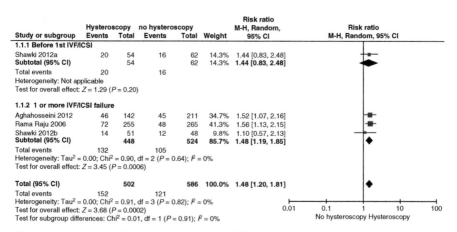

Women with previous implantation failure and women undergoing first IVF/ICSI attempt.
Hysteroscopy versus no hysteroscopy. Live birth rate

Fig. 4.8 Forest plot depicting the benefit in live birth rates by performing hysteroscopy both in women undergoing first IVF cycle and IVF performed after one or more failed cycle. Source: "Efficacy of hysteroscopy in improving reproductive outcomes of infertile couples: a systematic review and meta-analysis" by Sardo Atillo et al. 2016. Human Reprod Update; 22:479–496. Copyright 2016. Reproduced with permission from Oxford University Press

The concept of the "patient-tailored approach" and the increasing interest and clinical relevance in shortening time to pregnancy clearly explain why fertility specialists need to improve each single detail in order to improve patients' success rate in the least possible attempts. As a result, the scientific community has been rightly reconsidering the clinical relevance of hysteroscopy in the diagnosis and treatment of uterine factors, owing to its potential role of overcoming hidden undiagnosed uterine pathologies, capability to improve reproductive outcomes, and reducing time to pregnancy [1].

A screening hysteroscopy may turn out to be cost-effective, under the pretext of minimizing any negative anatomical intrauterine influence and hence increasing live births with hysteroscopy [30].

Hence, it is justified in not just an IVF program but also in low-risk patients before undergoing infertility treatment [35].

Women with high BMI (higher risk of endometrial polyps) and higher age (more prone for submucous myomas, endometrial hyperplasia, and polyps) especially should be preferred for hysteroscopy [39].

Amidst the often ongoing debate of usefulness of routine hysteroscopy as a baseline work-up tool in subfertile patients, the often used arguments against routine hysteroscopy are [35]:

1. Hysteroscopy is invasive.
2. Requires anesthesia (local or general).
3. Complications of possible intrauterine adhesions.

But recent medical advances have facilitated by allowing the invasiveness to be considerably reduced by decreasing size of scope (miniscope) and thereby allowing faster evaluation without anesthesia, dilatation, or sedation. Adhesions too are mostly preventable with balloon, barriers, high-dose estrogen [35].

Conclusion

The beneficial role of endoscopic evaluation of uterine environment cannot be emphasized enough. An increasing number of experimental and clinical studies distinctly recommend its success in improving spontaneous and post-ART fertility. Hysteroscopy should be performed in every patient who fails to conceive after replacement of good quality embryos at IVF and in any patient before entering IVF when a suspicion of intrauterine pathology arises from TVS/SSG/HSG. The possibility of a routine hysteroscopy before entering an IVF program should be seriously considered [20].

While debating the need for routine diagnostic hysteroscopy as a first-line evaluation tool of the infertile woman, it is helpful to remember that this procedure today is no longer a technically complicated or high-risk "in-patient general anesthesia one" but rather a simple, fast, low-risk outpatient procedure, requiring short training with proven high success rates [17].

The acceptance via successful implantation of a morphologically normal embryo in apparently good endometrium uterus remains the bottleneck in every IVF program. And hysteroscopy is a must to ensure there are no obvious missed in utero abnormalities.

References

1. Sardo AD, Carlo CD, Minozzi S, Spinelli M, Pistotti V, Alviggi C, et al. Efficacy of hysteroscopy in improving reproductive outcomes of infertile couples: a systematic review and meta-analysis. Hum Reprod Update. 2016;22:479–96.
2. The Practice Committee of the American Society for Reproductive Medicine. Definitions of infertility and recurrent pregnancy loss. Fertil Steril. 2008;90(Suppl):S60.
3. Templeton A, Morris JK, Parslow W. Factors that affect outcome of in-vitro fertilization treatment. Lancet. 1996;348:1402–6.
4. Kamphuis EI, Bhattacharya S, van der Veen F, Mol BW, Templeton A, Evidence Based IVF Group. Are we overusing IVF? BMJ. 2014;348:g252.
5. Ferraretti AP, Goossens V, de Mouzon J, et al. Assisted reproductive technology in Europe, 2008: results generated from European registers by ESHRE. Hum Reprod. 2012;27:2571–84.
6. Smit JG, Kasius JC, Eijkemans MJ, et al. Hysteroscopy before in-vitro fertilization (inSIGHT): a multicenter randomised controlled trial. Lancet. 2016;387:2622–9.
7. Andersen AN, Goossens V, Ferraretti AP, Bhattacharya S, Felberbaum R, de Mouzon J, et al. Assisted reproductive technology in Europe, 2004: results generated from European registers by ESHRE. Hum Reprod. 2008;23:756–71.
8. Bosteels J, Kasius J, Weyers S, Broekmans FJ, Mol BWJ, D'Hooghe TM. Hysteroscopy for treating subfertility associated with suspected major uterine cavity abnormalities. Cochrane Database Syst Rev. 2015;(2):CD009461. https://doi.org/10.1002/14651858.CD009461.pub3.
9. SEGI. Practical guideline in office hysteroscopy. 2014. Available at: http://ebookbrowsee.net/practical-guideline-in-office-hysteroscopy-segi-pdf-d715780654. Accessed on 5 May 2017.
10. Bettocchi S, Ceci O, Di Venere R, Pansini MV, Pellegrino A, Marello F, Nappi L. Advanced operative office hysteroscopy without anaesthesia: analysis of 501 cases treated with a 5 Fr. bipolar electrode. Hum Reprod. 2002;17:2435–8.
11. El-Toukhy T, Khalaf Y, Coomarasamy A et al. A multicenter randomised study of pre-IVF outpatient hysteroscopy in women with recurrent IVF-ET failure – the trophy trial. Oral communication, ESHRE 30th Annual Meeting. Munich, 2014.
12. Campo R, Meier R, Dhont N, Mestdagh G, Ombelet W. Implementation of hysteroscopy in an infertility clinic: the one-stop uterine diagnosis and treatment. Facts Views Vis Obgyn. 2014;6(4):235–9.
13. Pundir J, El-Toukhy T. Uterine cavity assessment prior to IVF. Womens Health. 2010;6:841–8.
14. Apirakviriya C, Rungruxsirivorn T, Phupong V, Wisawasukmongchol W. Diagnostic accuracy of 3D-transvaginal ultrasound in detecting uterine cavity abnormalities in infertile patients as compared with hysteroscopy. Eur J Obstet Gynecol Reprod Biol. 2016;200:24–8.
15. Wang CW, Lee CL, Lai YM, Tsai CC, Chang MY, Soong YK. Comparison of hysterosalpingography and hysteroscopy in female infertility. J Am Assoc Gynecol Laparosc. 1996;3(4):581–4.
16. Shushan A, Rojansky N. Should hysteroscopy be a part of the basic infertility workup? Hum Reprod. 1999;14(8):1923–4.
17. Pansky M, Feingold M, Sagi R, Herman A, Schneider D, Halperin R. Diagnostic hysteroscopy as a primary tool in a basic infertility workup. JSLS. 2006;10:231–5.
18. La Torre R, De Felice C, De Angelis C, Coacci F, Mastrone M, Cosmi EV. Transvaginal sonographic evaluation of endometrial polyps: a comparison with two dimensional and three dimensional contrast sonography. Clin Exp Obstet Gynecol. 1999;26:171–3.
19. Cunha-Filho JSL, de Souza CAB, Salazar CC, Facin AC, Freitas FM, Passos EP. Accuracy of hysterosalpingography and hysteroscopy for diagnosis of intrauterine lesions in infertile patients in an assisted fertilization program. Gynaecol Endosc. 2001;10(1):45–8.
20. Golan A, Ron-El R, Herman A, Soffer Y, Bukovsky I, Caspi E. Diagnostic hysteroscopy: its value in an in-vitro fertilization/embryo transfer unit. Hum Reprod. 1992;7(10):1433–4.
21. Radwan P, Radwan M, Polac I, Wilczynski JR. Detection of intracavitary lesions in 820 infertile women: comparison of outpatient hysteroscopy with histopathological examination. Ginekol Pol. 2013;84:857–61.

22. NICE. Fertility: assessment and treatment for people with fertility problems. National Institute for Health and Clinical Excellence, 2013. Available at: http://guidance.nice.org.uk/CG156. Accessed on 5 Feb 2017.
23. The Practice Committee of the American Society for Reproductive Medicine. Diagnostic evaluation of the infertile female: a committee opinion. Fertil Steril. 2012;98:302–7.
24. Campo R, Van Belle Y, Rombauts L, Brosens I, Gordts S. Office mini-hysteroscopy. Hum Reprod Update. 1999;5(1):73–81.
25. Stefanescu A, Marinescu B. Diagnostic hysteroscopy - a retrospective study of 1545 cases. Maedica. 2012;7:4.
26. Molinas CR, Campo R. Office hysteroscopy and adenomyosis. Best Pract Res Clin Obstet Gynaecol. 2006;20(4):557–67.
27. Pundir J, Pundir V, Omanwa K, Khalaf Y, El Toukhy T. Hysteroscopy prior to the first IVF cycle: a systematic review and meta-analysis. Reprod Biomed Online. 2014;28:151–61.
28. Mansour R, Aboulghar M. Optimizing the embryo transfer technique. Hum Reprod. 2000;17:1149–53.
29. Romero R, Espinoza J, Mazor M. Can endometrial infection/inflammation explain implantation failure, spontaneous abortion, and preterm birth after in vitro fertilization? Fertil Steril. 2004;82:799–804.
30. Kasius JC, Eijkemans RJ, Mol BW, Fauser BC, Fatemi HM, Broekmans FJ. Cost-effectiveness of hysteroscopy screening for infertile women. Reprod Biomed Online. 2013;26:619–26.
31. Mooney SB, Milki AA. Effect of hysteroscopy performed in the cycle preceding controlled ovarian hyperstimulation on the outcome of in vitro fertilization. Fertil Steril. 2003;79:637–8.
32. Gulumser C, Narvekar N, Pathak M, Palmer E, Parker S, Saridogan E. See-and-treat outpatient hysteroscopy: an analysis of 1109 examinations. Reprod Biomed Online. 2010;20:423–9.
33. De Placido G, Clarizia R, Cadente C, Castaldo G, Romano C, Mollo A, et al. Compliance and diagnostic efficacy of mini-hysteroscopy versus traditional hysteroscopy in infertility investigation. Eur J Obstet Gynecol Reprod Biol. 2007;135(1):83–7.
34. El Toukhy T. Outpatient hysteroscopy and subsequent IVF cycle outcome: a systematic review and metaanalysis. Reprod Biomed Online. 2008;16(5):712–9.
35. Nawroth F, Foth D. Hysteroscopy only after recurrent IVF failure? Reprod Biomed Online. 2004;8:726.
36. Royal College of Obstetricians and Gynecologists Evidence-based Clinical Guidelines. Guideline: fertility assessment and treatment for people with fertility problems, 2004. RCOG website http://www.rcog.org.uk. Accessed on 17 Feb 2017.
37. Crosignani PG, Rubin BL. Optimal use of infertility diagnostic tests and treatments. Hum Reprod. 2000;15:723–32.
38. Bosteels J, Weyers S, Puttemans P, Panayotidis C, Herendael BV, Gomel V, et al. The effectiveness of hysteroscopy in improving pregnancy rates in subfertile women without other gynecological symptoms: a systematic review. Hum Reprod Update. 2010;16(1):1–11.
39. HT Y, Wang CJ, Lee CL, Huang HY. The role of diagnostic hysteroscopy before the first in vitro fertilization/intracytoplasmic sperm injection cycle. Arch Gynecol Obstet. 2012;286(5):1323–8.

Polyps: Hysteroscopic Diagnosis and Management

Sangita Sharma

5.1 Introduction

Endometrial polyps are common in the women of reproductive age group, although might be encountered even after menopause. They are localized hyperplastic overgrowths, consisting of both the endometrial glands and stroma, which protrude from the surface of the endometrium into the uterine cavity [1, 2]. Sometimes, polyps can also be found in the endocervical canal. At times, the polyps may contain smooth muscle fibers also, and then they are known as adenomatous polyps [3]. They may be single or multiple and sessile or pedunculated and may range from few millimeters to centimeters in size [2, 4, 5].

5.2 Epidemiology

The actual incidence of endometrial polyps is not known due to its asymptomatic prevalence and variable presentation [6–10]. The reported prevalence of endometrial polyps in women varies widely and ranges from 7.8% to 34.9%, depending on the definition of a polyp, diagnostic method used, and the population studied [11–14]. Endometrial polyps can be found in about 24–41% women with abnormal uterine bleeding and in 10% of asymptomatic women [15, 16]. The prevalence of polyps has been found to be higher in infertile women [6].

S. Sharma, MD (OBGY), DNB, FNB (Reprod. Med.)
Manipal Fertility, Manipal Hospital, Jaipur, Rajasthan, India

© Springer Nature Singapore Pte Ltd. 2018
S. Jain, D. B. Inamdar (eds.), *Manual of Fertility Enhancing Hysteroscopy*,
https://doi.org/10.1007/978-981-10-8028-9_5

5.3   Etiology and Pathogenesis

Risk factors associated with the development of endometrial polyps are age, obesity, hypertension, diabetes, hormone replacement therapy (HRT), and tamoxifen use [17–21]. The knowledge about the natural history of polyps is limited as most of them are asymptomatic and thus remain undiagnosed. According to DeWaay et al., spontaneous regression of endometrial polyp happens in around 27% cases in 1 year follow-up [16]. Smaller polyps tend to regress more as compared to bigger ones [10, 16].

Endometrial polyps may progress to atypical hyperplasia or endometrial carcinoma in a small percentage of patients. Reported incidence of malignant change in polyps is 0–12.9% [14, 22–28].

5.4   Clinical Presentation

Many women having endometrial polyps remain asymptomatic [6]. Most of the polyps are diagnosed only as an incidental finding during a pelvic ultrasound for other indications [5]. Of all the premenopausal women with endometrial polyps, 64–88% are symptomatic [29], most commonly presenting with menorrhagia, irregular menses, postcoital bleeding, or intermenstrual bleeding—abnormal uterine bleeding being the commonest clinical presentation [6]. Abnormal uterine bleeding due to polyp has been classified as AUB-P for premenopausal women by FIGO [30]. In women suffering from premenopausal bleeding, polyps are found in 10–40% of them [14, 15, 31]. Symptoms generally do not correlate with the number, size, or location of the polyp [32]. Fifty-six percent of postmenopausal women with polyps are symptomatic, most common symptom being postmenopausal bleeding [29, 32].

5.4.1   Endometrial Polyps and Infertility

Endometrial polyps are associated with infertility, although the causal relationship is not yet established [33]. The hypothesized mechanisms are:

– Mechanical interference with sperm transportation and embryo implantation [1, 34]
– Defective implantation at the polyp site [3]
– Glands and stroma of the polyp being unresponsive to progesterone [3]
– Local inflammatory changes [35–37] and altered expression of the molecular markers of endometrial receptivity [1, 5, 38]

Higher levels of estrogen during controlled ovarian stimulation with gonadotropins increase risk of endometrial polyps [39]. The presence of endometrial polyps varies in women with infertility; in primary infertility, it was reported from 3.8% to

38.5%, whereas in secondary infertility it was found from 1.8% to 17% [33, 40–42]. This wide variation is due to the differences in the studied population and the diagnostic modalities used. Although this high prevalence of polyps in women with infertility indicates some kind of causal relationship [6], it has been proven only in one randomized trial [43].

5.5   Diagnosis

The common modalities used for diagnosis of endometrial polyp include two-dimensional transvaginal sonography (2D TVUS), three-dimensional transvaginal sonography (3D TVUS), saline infusion sonography (SIS), hysterosalpingography (HSG), and hysteroscopy [44].

2D TVUS can detect most of the endometrial polyps accurately and should be the investigation of choice (Level B) [6]. Polyps are better seen with 2D TVUS when assessed in mid-cycle. On adding color flow Doppler, the diagnostic capability of 2D TVUS can improve as it allows the visualization of the feeding vessel present in endometrial polyps [6]. 3D TVUS allows for the measurement of the endometrial volume, as well as the endometrial and sub-endometrial vascularization indices, but data comparing 2D TVUS and 3D TVUS for diagnosing endometrial polyps is conflicting [45, 46]. Saline infusion sonography (SIS) is a safe, rapid, and well-tolerated diagnostic method with good sensitivity [47]. It is better than transvaginal ultrasound for diagnosing endometrial polyps [48].

Hysterosalpingography (HSG) is more sensitive (98%), but less specific (34.6%) for diagnosing endometrial polyps, when compared to hysteroscopy [42, 49]. As it leads to patient discomfort and it involves use of iodine-containing radiopaque dyes with radiation, HSG is not much preferred for this indication.

Magnetic resonance imaging (MRI) has limited advantages over sonography for diagnosing endometrial polyps and is also restricted by the high cost and limited availability. Computed tomography scanning also has a low sensitivity (53%) in comparison to transvaginal ultrasound [50].

Hysteroscopy is the gold standard for the diagnosis of endometrial polyps [6, 51], and it is the only modality which offers an opportunity for concurrent treatment. Simultaneous assessment of the size, number, vascular characteristics, and other features of endometrial polyps (sessile or pedunculated) can also be done (Figs. 5.1 and 5.2) [6]. Blind dilation and curettage should not be used for the diagnosis of endometrial polyps [6] as it can cause polyp fragmentation making histopathologic diagnosis difficult [52, 53]. Blind endometrial sampling also has a low sensitivity (8–46%) and low NPV (7–58%) as compared to hysteroscopy with guided biopsy [54].

Hysteroscopic-guided biopsy is the most sensitive and highly specific method for diagnosing an endometrial polyp, and therefore other techniques are most commonly compared with it [55]. If diagnostic hysteroscopy is done alone, without a guided biopsy, it permits only a visual assessment of the size and type of the lesion, with a reported sensitivity of 58–99%, specificity of 87–100%, PPV of 21–100%,

Fig. 5.1 A pedunculated
vascular endometrial polyp
on hysteroscopy

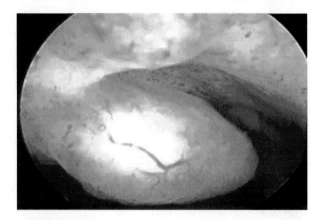

Fig. 5.2 A sessile polyp
on the anterior wall of the
cavity

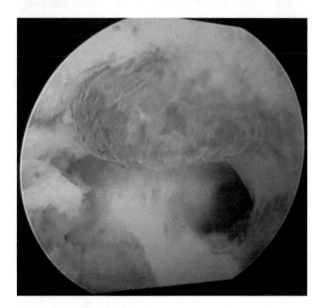

and NPV of 66–99% [13, 51, 56–59]. The hysteroscopy (diagnostic as well as therapeutic) can be done as an outpatient or inpatient procedure, depending on availability of instruments, patient's preference, and expertise of the operator [51, 60, 61].

5.6   Management of Endometrial Polyps

Nowadays with the higher resolution of ultrasound machines and the increasing use
of ultrasound as a primary tool for gynecological conditions, the diagnosis of endometrial polyps as an incidental finding is increasing. This results in dilemma to the
gynecologists, especially regarding the management of asymptomatic and incidental endometrial polyps.

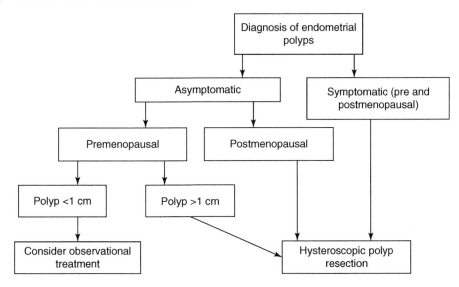

Fig. 5.3 Suggested treatment algorithm for women with endometrial polyps. Source: "The management of endometrial polyps in the 21st century," by John Jude Annan et al. 2012, The Obstetrician & Gynecologist, 14, pp. 33–38. Copyright 2012 Reproduced with permission from John Wiley and Sons

5.6.1   Expectant Management

Since the natural course of endometrial polyps is not well understood [11, 16] and most of the polyps are benign, expectant management seems to be a reasonable option, especially in women who are asymptomatic and premenopausal and when the polyp size is <10 mm [6]. Small endometrial polyps (<10 mm) are thought to regress spontaneously in about 25% of cases [62, 63].

Figure 5.3 shows a suggested treatment algorithm for women with endometrial polyps based on the current evidence [64].

5.6.2   Medical Management

There is no role of medical management in endometrial polyps associated with infertility [6, 63]. Levonorgestrel-containing intrauterine devices have been used to prevent tamoxifen-related endometrial polyps, but its use for treatment of polyps should be currently limited to research protocols [65].

5.6.3   Surgical Management

Although most of the polyps, especially the smaller ones, might regress spontaneously, definitive treatment options are mainly surgical.

1. **Blind Dilation and Curettage**: Blind dilatation and curettage should be avoided as endometrial pathology can be missed in about 50% cases [52–54].
2. **Hysteroscopic Resection of Polyps**: Hysteroscopic resection is considered gold standard in surgical management of polyps. It is safe and effective and has the advantage of both diagnosis and treatment in the same sitting and additional advantage of obtaining tissue for histopathologic diagnosis [6].

5.7 Hysteroscopic Resection of Polyps

5.7.1 Procedure

Hysteroscopic polypectomy, like any other operative hysteroscopy, is preferably scheduled in the postmenstrual phase. Ongoing pregnancy, malignancy, and active gynecological infection should be ruled out before any hysteroscopic procedure. It is best performed in dorsal lithotomy position under aseptic conditions after perineal and vaginal cleaning with 10% betadine solution.

As the incidence of postoperative infection is low, routine antibiotic prophylaxis is not needed [66, 67]. But as fertility might be compromised after an episode of postoperative endometritis, some authors have supported the use of antibiotics after complex operative hysteroscopic procedures like myomectomy, septum resection, or lysis of synechiae. The preferred antibiotics are a cephalosporin or doxycycline [66].

Usually an initial per speculum inspection of the cervix and a bimanual per vaginum examination are done before proceeding with hysteroscopy, the exception being the vaginoscopic approach, where these are omitted (*vide infra*). This is followed by progressive dilatation of the cervix, if required, depending on the diameter of the operative hysteroscope being used. After checking the assembly of the instruments, the flow of distension medium is started, and the hysteroscope is introduced in the cervical canal. The cervical canal should be visualized to proceed in the right direction and also to rule out any pathology or lesion. After crossing the internal os and entering the uterine cavity, a few seconds are given for the distension of the cavity by the distension medium to have a clear view. A complete evaluation should be done including all the walls of the uterine cavity, the fundus, the tubal ostia, and the appearance of the endometrium. The polyps should be assessed in terms of size, number, location, vascularity, and sessile or pedunculated base. The surrounding endometrium should also be seen in detail. Depending on all these factors and the availability of the instruments, one can choose the hysteroscopic instrument to be used for polypectomy.

In the vaginoscopic approach to hysteroscopy, there is no need of speculum and tenaculum, resulting in lesser pain [68]. The results of polypectomy are comparable [69].

Inability to perform outpatient hysteroscopy is mostly due to technical difficulty related to anatomical factors (e.g., cervical stenosis), improper visualization, and patient intolerance [70].

5.7.2   Office Hysteroscopy vs. Inpatient Procedure

As already mentioned, hysteroscopy can be done both as an outdoor and an indoor procedure, based on patient preference, instrument availability, the choice of the surgeon, and the size and location of the polyps [6, 71]. Office hysteroscopy has become popular nowadays, but still a large number of routine diagnostic hysteroscopies are still performed under general anesthesia after hospitalization [51, 61]. The results of outpatient hysteroscopy for diagnosis of endometrial polyps are encouraging, both in premenopausal and postmenopausal women [31, 51]. It is reported to be less expensive with greater patient comfort [72]. Removal of small polyps is also possible; however, failure to perform a polypectomy has also been reported [71]. Office-based hysteroscopic polypectomy is safe and feasible in patients with endometrial or isthmic polyps ≤20 mm, independent of menopausal status or previous vaginal delivery [73]. Thus office hysteroscopy is cost-effective and gives more patient comfort but requires a high level of expertise, especially if an operative procedure is required simultaneously. The use of paracervical block may be helpful, particularly in operative hysteroscopy [74]. Technological improvements and the availability of narrow-diameter hysteroscopes have made operative hysteroscopy easier as an outpatient procedure [60].

5.7.3   Flexible vs. Rigid Hysteroscopy

As compared to rigid hysteroscopy, flexible hysteroscopy permits a smoother entry through the cervical canal and thus causes less pain to the patient [75, 76]. Thus, it is better suited for outdoor procedures. It has a lower sensitivity of 74% for detecting endometrial polyps, compared to rigid hysteroscopy [77, 78]. The drawbacks of flexible hysteroscopes are the higher cost, instrument delicacy with more chances of breakage, and limited operative instrumentation.

Table 5.1 summarizes the different methods and techniques practiced to remove polyps at hysteroscopy with their relative advantages and disadvantages.

5.7.4   Type of Instruments Used for Polypectomy

Different hysteroscopic systems and instruments have been used for hysteroscopic removal of polyps. These include hysteroscopic microscissors or graspers [6], resectoscope with monopolar loop cautery [6], bipolar resectoscope [29, 85], and hysteroscopic morcellators [83, 84].

The choice of instrument is based on the cost, availability, size, and location of the polyp and operator's expertise. A few studies comparing the abovementioned methods with regard to cost and efficacy have been reported.

Small and pedunculated polyps are easily removed either with **scissors** or **small polyp forceps** through the operating hysteroscope (Figs. 5.4, 5.5, and 5.6) [80]. The grasping forceps should be directed at the base of the polyp, and rather than pulling,

Table 5.1 Different methods and techniques for removal of polyps [79]

Management	Advantages	Disadvantages	Recurrence
Dilatation and curettage or hysteroscopy followed by blind grasping forceps/curettage [54, 80]	Readily available Low equipment costs Minimal expertise required	Low sensitivity (8–46%) General anesthesia Hospitalization required Complication rates higher than with targeted removal	Recurrence in 15%
Hysteroscopic polypectomy [60, 75, 80–82]	Accurate, complete resection of polyp Early recovery, return to normal activities Minimal hospitalization Low risk of complication (0.38%) Associated with good reproductive outcome Low risk of intrauterine adhesions with operative hysteroscopy for polyps	Increased operating time for operative hysteroscopy Specialized equipment Glycine absorption and associated complications are potential issues Higher skill requirement than blind technique	Operative hysteroscope use is associated with a low recurrence rate of 0–4.5%
Hysteroscopy and polyp morcellation [83, 84]	Easy to use No glycine for distension Timesaving Short learning curve	Expensive Not widely available Increased difficulty of pathological examination Increased risk of bleeding as no electrosurgery	Not yet reported
Hysteroscopy and bipolar removal of polyp [29, 85]	Easy to use No glycine for distension	Expensive Not widely available	Not yet reported
Hysterectomy	Definitive treatment No risk for future malignancy Treatment of choice for polyp	High risk of surgical morbidity Compromises future childbearing ability	No recurrence
Medical	Noninvasive	Only for short-term treatment Limited evidence of effectiveness	Symptom recurrence on treatment cessation

Fig. 5.4 Hysteroscope (2.9 mm) with diagnostic and operative sheaths

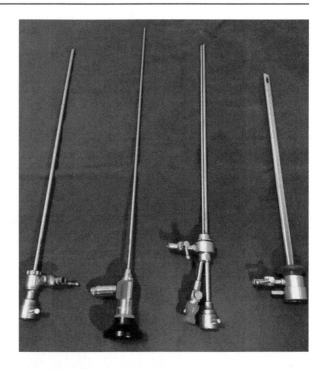

Fig. 5.5 Hysteroscope with assembled operative sheath and hysteroscopic scissors

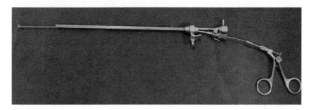

Fig. 5.6 Tip of hystero-scopic scissors

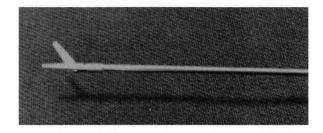

a gentle but consistent forward pressure is maintained to avulse the polyp from its base. The polyp is then removed through the hysteroscope along with the grasper. The polyp can be removed in one or more attempts according to its size.

On the other hand, electrosurgical loop (resectoscope) is the instrument of choice for large and sessile polyps (Figs. 5.7 and 5.8). Once the concerned polyp is brought in good view, the resectoscope loop is advanced and taken beyond the polyp. After

Fig. 5.7 Monopolar
resectoscope with
electrosurgical loop and
sheaths

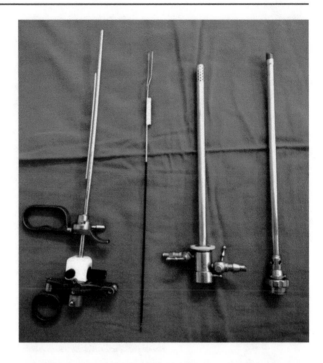

Fig. 5.8 Electrosurgical
loop for polypectomy

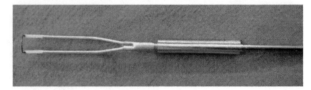

this the foot pedal or hand control is used to switch on the flow of the current
through the loop, and it is simultaneously pulled proximally in the direction away
from the fundus. Multiple such repetitive attempts are made as the broad-based
polyp is shaved in piecemeal. The *resectoscopic polypectomy* may take longer operating time which can lead to complications due to systemic glycine absorption. The
chances of recurrence are almost nil when compared to other methods such as
microscissors or grasping forceps (15%) [80].

Bipolar electrosurgical resection systems [(Bipolar Versapoint (Gynecare,
Sommerville, NJ) or Gynecare Versascope™ (ETHICON TM)] are thinner instruments which require minimal cervical dilatation. They are compatible with saline as
distension medium, thus decreasing the risk of hyponatremia and its sequel [29, 85].
Bipolar twizzles [86] and polyp snares [87] have shown good success and low pain
scores. Bipolar electrode excision is better for small, fundal polyps, while monopolar excision is preferable for nonfundal polyps or the larger ones (>20 mm) [88].

The hysteroscopic morcellator enables simultaneous removal of pieces of polyp
as it resects under direct vision in a shorter time. There is no need for repeated in and

out movement of instrument, hence less chances of fluid loss and cervical trauma [84]. Traditionally, polyps >2 cm or those larger than the diameter of the internal cervical os are best removed with the patient under general anesthesia as there is a longer operating time, increased patient discomfort, passage of instruments multiple times through the cervix, and piecemeal removal of the polyp. Morcellators with lesser diameters are becoming available for such a situation. An added advantage is the ease with which multiple polyps can be removed. In a randomized study of 121 patients, removal of polyps using a hysteroscopic morcellator was found to be significantly quicker, less painful, more acceptable to women, and more likely to completely remove endometrial polyps compared to electrosurgical resection [89].

Bipolar electrosurgical resection and hysteroscopic morcellation are the techniques which are expensive and not available widely. At present there is limited evidence about their efficacy in improving reproductive outcome. More randomized trials are needed before reaching a conclusion.

5.7.5 Complications of Hysteroscopic Polypectomy

Hysteroscopic polypectomy is a safe procedure with a reported complication rate of 0.95–3% [81, 90, 91]. The most common complications for operative hysteroscopy are:

- Hemorrhage (2.4%)
- Perforation of the uterus (1.5%)
- Cervical laceration (1–11%) [91]
- Complications due to excessive fluid absorption like hyponatremia, etc. [81, 90–92]

However, most of these complications are associated with prolonged operative hysteroscopy like adhesiolysis and myomectomy and less commonly encountered with polypectomy.

Hemorrhage can be seen either during or after hysteroscopy. In case of excess bleeding, uterine perforation should be ruled out. Mild hemorrhage generally stops on its own and does not require any specific intervention. In case of moderate to severe bleeding, electrocautery can be used to coagulate small vessels. If the bleeding is still not controlled, a Foley catheter or intrauterine balloon can be inserted and inflated in the cavity for a tamponade effect [92, 93].

Uterine perforation is one of the common complications of operative hysteroscopy, the incidence being 0.7–3%. The perforation can occur through introduction of uterine sound, cervical dilator, hysteroscope, or any other operative instrument like hysteroscopic scissors, a morcellator, or a resectoscope cautery loop. The surgeon should counsel and take a written consent from all the patients beforehand regarding the possible complications and for a simultaneous laparoscopy if required [81, 90, 91]. A small perforation with a blunt instrument can be managed conservatively, but if suspected with a sharp instrument or an electrocautery loop, a concurrent laparoscopy should be done to rule out injury to the pelvis viscera or vessels.

The risk of intrauterine adhesions is low as the myometrium is generally not incised [94]. No adhesions were reported after hysteroscopic polypectomy in a class 1 study [82]. Other less common complications associated with the procedure include anesthesia-related complications, formation of a false passage in the cervical canal, postoperative endometritis, and rarely gas embolism. The complications are discussed further in detail elsewhere in this book.

5.7.6 American Association of Gynecologic Laparoscopists (AAGL) Guidelines for the Management of Endometrial Polyps [6]

1. Conservative management is reasonable, particularly for small polyps and if asymptomatic (Level A).
2. Medical management of polyps cannot be recommended (Level B).
3. Hysteroscopic polypectomy remains the gold standard for treatment (Level B).
4. No difference in clinical outcomes with various hysteroscopic polypectomy techniques (Level C).
5. Removal for histologic assessment is appropriate in postmenopausal women with symptoms (Level B).
6. Hysteroscopic removal is to be preferred to hysterectomy because of its less invasive nature, lower cost, and reduced risk to the patient (Level C).

For the infertile patient with a polyp, surgical removal is recommended to allow natural conception or assisted reproductive technology a greater opportunity to be successful (Level A).

5.8 Role of Polypectomy in Conception

5.8.1 Natural Conception

A few observational studies have shown improvement in natural conception rates after resection of endometrial polyps, particularly in patients with unexplained infertility [1, 95]. In a study of 266 infertile, eumenorrheic women, a pregnancy rate of 50% was achieved following hysteroscopic polypectomy [34]. According to present evidence, polypectomy is effective in improving pregnancy rates in subfertile women (43–80%) [36, 80, 96].

5.8.2 Intrauterine Insemination

Polypectomy increases conception rate in patients undergoing intrauterine insemination (IUI) [5, 43]. In a prospective study, 86 women underwent hysteroscopic polypectomy before IUI, and 85 women opted to proceed directly with IUI without polyp removal. On comparison, pregnancy rates were 40.7% after polypectomy as compared to 22.3% in controls [97]. According to recent Cochrane systematic review, hysteroscopic removal of polyps prior to IUI increases the odds of clinical pregnancy compared to diagnostic hysteroscopy and polyp biopsy alone (OR 4.4, 95% CI 2.5–8.0 and $p < 0.00001$) [95].

5.8.3 In Vitro Fertilization

According to a systematic review, if polyps are detected before the start of controlled ovarian hyperstimulation, they should be removed to improve the outcome of IVF [35]. The management of newly diagnosed endometrial polyps during ovarian stimulation still remains controversial [1, 5]. Management of polyps which appear during the ovarian stimulation should be customized based on the number of embryos, history of previous conception, and robustness of cryopreservation program of the respective center [35].

In a retrospective analysis of 83 patients which were suspected to have endometrial polyps of <2 cm on TVUS, similar pregnancy rate was found whether fresh embryo transfer was done or it was frozen embryo transfer after hysteroscopic polypectomy, but miscarriage rate was significantly higher in the fresh transfer group. So polypectomy can increase the take-home baby rates by reducing miscarriage rate [98].

In another retrospective analysis, it was found that endometrial polyps <1.5 cm, seen during ovarian stimulation, did not require removal. The pregnancy and live birth rates were similar in patients diagnosed with an endometrial polyp (when compared to controls) in ICSI cycles. Thus it was concluded that such polyps can be managed expectantly [99].

Retrospective study by Check et al. showed no difference in the implantation, clinical pregnancy, or live birth rates after fresh IVF-ET cycles when patients with newly diagnosed endometrial polyps were compared to those without polyp [100].

In a recent retrospective cohort study, it was concluded that newly diagnosed endometrial polyps during COH are associated with an increased biochemical pregnancy rate (odds ratio, 2.12; 95% CI, 1.09–4.12) but ultimately do not adversely impact clinical pregnancy or live birth rates after fresh IVF-ET [5].

In a subset of patients with recurrent implantation failure in IVF cycles, there was a significant increase in implantation and clinical pregnancy rates subsequent to hysteroscopic removal of endometrial polyps [101].

The time interval between hysteroscopic polypectomy and the subsequent IVF cycle does not seem to impact the success rates of the IVF cycle [102].

In conclusion, surgical resection of endometrial polyps is recommended in infertile patients to possibly increase natural conception rates, as well as those associated with assisted reproductive technology [6]. Management of newly diagnosed endometrial polyps during IVF should be individualized [5, 35].

Conclusion

1. The prevalence of endometrial polyps is higher in infertile women.
2. Hysteroscopy is the gold standard for the diagnosis of endometrial polyps and is the only modality which offers an opportunity for concurrent treatment.
3. Office hysteroscopy is cost-effective and gives more patient comfort but requires a high level of expertise, especially if an operative procedure is required simultaneously.
4. There is no evidence to favor any one hysteroscopic polypectomy technique over the others in terms of clinical outcome.
5. Hysteroscopic polypectomy is indicated for polyps associated with infertility.
6. Resection of endometrial polyps, particularly in patients with unexplained infertility, improves natural conception rates and conception rates with IUI.
7. Polyps diagnosed prior to commencement of controlled ovarian hyperstimulation (COH) for in vitro fertilization (IVF) should be removed.
8. Management of newly diagnosed endometrial polyps during IVF should be individualized.

References

1. Taylor E, Gomel V. The uterus and fertility. Fertil Steril. 2008;89(1):1–16.
2. Rackow BW, Jorgensen E, Taylor HS. Endometrial polyps affect uterine receptivity. Fertil Steril. 2011;95(8):2690–2.
3. Mittal K, Schwartz L, Goswami S, Demopoulos R. Estrogen and progesterone receptor expression in endometrial polyps. Int J Gynecol Pathol. 1996;15(4):345–8.
4. Kim KR, Peng R, Ro JY, Robboy SJ. A diagnostically useful histopathologic feature of endometrial polyp: the long axis of endometrial glands arranged parallel to surface epithelium. Am J Surg Pathol. 2004;28:1057–62.
5. Elias RT, Pereira N, Karipcin FS, Rosenwaks Z, Spandorfer SD. Impact of newly diagnosed endometrial polyps during controlled ovarian hyperstimulation on in vitro fertilization outcomes. J Minim Invasive Gynecol. 2015;22(4):590–4.
6. American Association of Gynecologic Laparoscopists. AAGL practice report: practice guidelines for the diagnosis and management of endometrial polyps. J Minim Invasive Gynecol. 2012;19(1):3–10.
7. Fay TN, Khanem N, Hosking D. Out-patient hysteroscopy in asymptomatic postmenopausal women. Climacteric. 1999;2:263–7.
8. de Ziegler D. Contrast ultrasound: a simple-to-use phase-shifting medium offers saline infusion sonography-like images. Fertil Steril. 2009;92:369–73.
9. Martinez-Perez O, Perez-Medina T, Bajo-Arenas J. Ultrasonography of endometrial polyps. Ultrasound Rev Obstet Gynecol. 2003;3:43.
10. Lieng M, Istre O, Sandvik L, Qvigstad E. Prevalence, 1-year regression rate, and clinical significance of asymptomatic endometrial polyps: cross-sectional study. J Minim Invasive Gynecol. 2009;16:465–71.
11. Haimov-Kochman R, Deri-Hasid R, Hamani Y, Voss E. The natural course of endometrial polyps: could they vanish when left untreated? Fertil Steril. 2009;92:828.e11–2.
12. Dreisler E, Stampe Sorensen S, Ibsen PH, Lose G. Prevalence of endometrial polyps and abnormal uterine bleeding in a Danish population aged 20-74 years. Ultrasound Obstet Gynecol. 2009;33:102–8.

13. Fabres C, Alam V, Balmaceda J, Zegers-Hochschild F, Mackenna A, Fernandez E. Comparison of ultrasonography and hysteroscopy in the diagnosis of intrauterine lesions in infertile women. J Am Assoc Gynecol Laparosc. 1998;5:375–8.
14. Anastasiadis PG, Koutlaki NG, Skaphida PG, Galazios GC, Tsikouras PN, Liberis VA. Endometrial polyps: prevalence, detection, and malignant potential in women with abnormal uterine bleeding. Eur J Gynaecol Oncol. 2000;21:180–3.
15. Clevenger-Hoeft M, Syrop C, Stovall D, Van Voorhis B. Sonohysterography in premenopausal women with and without abnormal bleeding. Obstet Gynecol. 1999;94:516–20.
16. DeWaay DJ, Syrop CH, Nygaard IE, Davis WA, Van Voorhis BJ. Natural history of uterine polyps and leiomyomata. Obstet Gynecol. 2002;100:3–7.
17. Cohen I. Endometrial pathologies associated with postmenopausal tamoxifen treatment. Gynecol Oncol. 2004;94:256–66.
18. Onalan R, Onalan G, Tonguc E, Ozdener T, Dogan M, Mollamahmutoglu L. Body mass index is an independent risk factor for the development of endometrial polyps in patients undergoing in vitro fertilization. Fertil Steril. 2009;91:1056–60.
19. Nappi L, Indraccolo U, Sardo ADS, et al. Are diabetes, hypertension, and obesity independent risk factors for endometrial polyps? J Minim Invasive Gynecol. 2009;16(2):157–62.
20. Dreisler E, Sorensen S, Lose G. Endometrial polyps and associated factors in Danish women aged 36–74 years. Am J Obstet Gynecol. 2009;200:e1–6.
21. Maia H Jr, Barbosa IC, Marques D, Calmon LC, Ladipo OA, Coutinho EM. Hysteroscopy and transvaginal sonography in menopausal women receiving hormone replacement therapy. J Am Assoc Gynecol Laparosc. 1996;4:13–8.
22. Bakour SH, Khan KS, Gupta JK. The risk of premalignant and malignant pathology in endometrial polyps. Acta Obstet Gynecol Scand. 2000;79:317–20.
23. Ben-Arie A, Goldchmit C, Laviv Y, et al. The malignant potential of endometrial polyps. Eur J Obstet Gynecol Reprod Biol. 2004;115:206–10.
24. Ferrazzi E, Zupi E, Leone FP, et al. How often are endometrial polyps malignant in asymptomatic postmenopausal women? A multicenter study. Am J Obstet Gynecol. 2009;200:235. e1–6.
25. Lieng M, Qvigstad E, Sandvik L, Jørgensen H, Langebrekke A, Istre O. Hysteroscopic resection of symptomatic and asymptomatic endometrial polyps. J Minim Invasive Gynecol. 2007;14:189–94.
26. Papadia A, Gerbaldo D, Fulcheri E, et al. The risk of premalignant and malignant pathology in endometrial polyps: should every polyp be resected? Minerva Ginecol. 2007;59:117–24.
27. Savelli L, De Iaco P, Santini D, et al. Histopathologic features and risk factors for benignity, hyperplasia, and cancer in endometrial polyps. Am J Obstet Gynecol. 2003;188:927–31.
28. Hileeto D, Fadare O, Martel M, Zheng W. Age dependent association of endometrial polyps with increased risk of cancer involvement. World J Surg Oncol. 2005;3:8.
29. Golan A, Sagiv R, Berar M, Ginath S, Glezerman M. Bipolar electrical energy in physiologic solution - a revolution in operative hysteroscopy. J Am Assoc Gynecol Laparosc. 2001;8:252–8.
30. Munro M, Critchley HO, Broder MS, Fraser IS. FIGO Working Group on Menstrual Disorders. FIGO classification system (PALM-COEIN) for causes of abnormal uterine bleeding in nongravid women of reproductive age. Int J Gynecol Obstet. 2011;113:3–11.
31. Nagele F, O'Connor H, Davies A, Badawy A, Mohamed H, Magos A. 2500 Outpatient diagnostic hysteroscopies. Obstet Gynecol. 1996;88:87–92.
32. Hassa H, Tekin B, Senses T, Kaya M, Karatas A. Are the site, diameter, and number of endometrial polyps related with symptomatology? Am J Obstet Gynecol. 2006;194:718–21.
33. Taylor P, Pattinson H, Kredenster J. Diagnostic hysteroscopy. In: Hunt R, editor. Atlas of female infertility. Boston, MA: Mosby–Year Book; 1992. p. 200.
34. Shokeir TA, Shalan HM, El-Shafei MM. Significance of endometrial polyps detected hysteroscopically in eumenorrheic infertile women. J Obstet Gynaecol Res. 2004;30:84–9.
35. Afifi K, Anand S, Nallapeta S, Gelbaya TA. Management of endometrial polyps in subfertile women: a systematic review. Eur J Obstet Gynecol Reprod Biol. 2010;151(2):117–21.

36. Spiewankiewicz B, Stelmachów J, Sawicki W, Cendrowski K, Wypych P, Swiderska K. The effectiveness of hysteroscopic polypectomy in cases of female infertility. Clin Exp Obstet Gynecol. 2003;30(1):23–5.
37. Al-Jefout M, Black K, Schulke L, et al. Novel finding of high density of activated mast cells in endometrial polyps. Fertil Steril. 2009;92(3):1104–6.
38. Richlin SS, Ramachandran S, Shanti A, Murphy AA, Parthasarathy S. Glycodelin levels in uterine flushings and in plasma of patients with leiomyomas and polyps: implications for implantation. Hum Reprod. 2002;17(10):2742–7.
39. Hinckley MD, Milki AA. 1000 office-based hysteroscopies prior to in vitro fertilization: feasibility and findings. JSLS. 2004;8:103–7.
40. Kupesic S, Kurjak A, Skenderovic S, Bjelos D. Screening for uterine abnormalities by three-dimensional ultrasound improves perinatal outcome. J Perinat Med. 2002;30:9–17.
41. Valle RF. Hysteroscopy in the evaluation of female infertility. Am J Obstet Gynecol. 1980;137:425–31.
42. Preutthipan S, Linasmita V. A prospective comparative study between hysterosalpingography and hysteroscopy in the detection of intrauterine pathology in patients with infertility. J Obstet Gynaecol Res. 2003;29:33–7.
43. Perez-Medina T, Bajo-Arenas J, Salazar F, et al. Endometrial polyps and their implication in the pregnancy rates of patients undergoing intrauterine insemination: a prospective, randomized study. Hum Reprod. 2005;20:1632–5.
44. Seshadri S, El-Toukhy T, Douiri A, Jayaprakasan K, Khalaf Y. Diagnostic accuracy of saline infusion sonography in the evaluation of uterine cavity abnormalities prior to assisted reproductive techniques: a systematic review and metaanalyses. Hum Reprod Update. 2015;21(2):262–74.
45. Fang L, Su Y, Guo Y, Sun Y. Value of 3-dimensional and power Doppler sonography for diagnosis of endometrial polyps. J Ultrasound Med. 2013;32(2):247–55.
46. La Torre R, De Felice C, De Angelis C, Coacci F, Mastrone M, Cosmi EV. Transvaginal sonographic evaluation of endometrial polyps: a comparison with two dimensional and three dimensional contrast sonography. Clin Exp Obstet Gynecol. 1999;26(3-4):171–3.
47. Guven MA, Bese T, Demirkiran F, Idil M, Mgoyi L. Hydrosonography in screening for intracavitary pathology in infertile women. Int J Gynaecol Obstet. 2004;86:377–83.
48. Kamel HS, Darwish AM, Mohamed SA. Comparison of transvaginal ultrasonography and vaginal sonohysterography in the detection of endometrial polyps. Acta Obstet Gynecol Scand. 2000;79:60–4.
49. Soares SR, Dos Reis MB, Camargos AF. Diagnostic accuracy of sonohysterography, transvaginal sonography, and hysterosalpingography in patients with uterine cavity diseases. Fertil Steril. 2000;73(2):406–11.
50. Grossman J, Ricci ZJ, Rozenblit A, Freeman K, Mazzariol F, Stein MW. Efficacy of contrast-enhanced CT in assessing the endometrium. AJR Am J Roentgenol. 2008;191:664–9.
51. Lo KWK, Yuen PM. The role of outpatient diagnostic hysteroscopy in identifying anatomic pathology and histopathology in the endometrial cavity. J Am Assoc Gynecol Laparosc. 2000;7(3):381–5.
52. Gimpelson RJ, Rappold HO. A comparative study between panoramic hysteroscopy with directed biopsies and dilatation and curettage. A review of 276 cases. Am J Obstet Gynecol. 1988;158(3):489–92.
53. Svirsky R, Smorgick N, Rozowski U, et al. Can we rely on blind endometrial biopsy for detection of focal intrauterine pathology? Am J Obstet Gynecol. 2008;199(2):115.e1–3.
54. Bettocchi S, Ceci O, Vicino M, Marello F, Impedovo L, Selvaggi L. Diagnostic inadequacy of dilatation and curettage. Fertil Steril. 2001;75(4):803–5.
55. Makris N, Kalmantis K, Skartados N, Papadimitriou A, Mantzaris G, Antsaklis A. Three-dimensional hysterosonography versus hysteroscopy for the detection of intracavitary uterine abnormalities. Int J Gynecol Obstet. 2007;97:6–9.
56. Schwärzler P, Concin H, Bösch H, Berlinger A, Wohlgenannt K, Collins WP, Bourne TH. An evaluation of sonohysterography and diagnostic hysteroscopy for the assessment of intrauterine pathology. Ultrasound Obstet Gynecol. 1998;11:337–42.

57. Pasqualotto EB, Margossian H, Price LL, Bradley LD. Accuracy of preoperative diagnostic tools and outcome of hysteroscopic management of menstrual dysfunction. J Am Assoc Gynecol Laparosc. 2000;7:201–9.
58. Makris N, Skartados N, Kalmantis K, Mantzaris G, Papadimitriou A, Antsaklis A. Evaluation of abnormal uterine bleeding by transvaginal 3-D hysterosonography and diagnostic hysteroscopy. Eur J Gynaecol Oncol. 2007;28:39–42.
59. Birinyi L, Daragó P, Török P, et al. Predictive value of hysteroscopic examination in intrauterine abnormalities. Eur J Obstet Gynecol Reprod Biol. 2004;115:75–9.
60. Bettocchi S, Ceci O, Nappi L, et al. Operative office hysteroscopy without anesthesia: analysis of 4863 cases performed with mechanical instruments. J Am Assoc Gynecol Laparosc. 2004;11:59–61.
61. Clark TJ, Khan KS, Gupta JK. Current practice for the treatment of benign intrauterine polyps: a national questionnaire survey of consultant gynaecologists in UK. Eur J Obstet Gynecol Reprod Biol. 2002;103:65–7.
62. Hamani Y, Eldar I, Sela HY, Voss E, Haimov-Kochman R. The clinical significance of small endometrial polyps. Eur J Obstet Gynecol Reprod Biol. 2013;170(2):497–500.
63. Lieng M, Istre O, Qvigstad E. Treatment of endometrial polyps: a systematic review. Acta Obstet Gynecol Scand. 2010;89(8):992–1002.
64. Annan JJ, Aquilina J, Ball E. The management of endometrial polyps in the 21st century. Obstet Gynaecol. 2012;14:33–8.
65. Gardner FJE, Konje JC, Bell SC, et al. Prevention of tamoxifen induced endometrial polyps using a levonorgestrel releasing intrauterine system. Long-term follow-up of a randomized control trial. Gynecol Oncol. 2009;114(3):452–6.
66. ACOG practice bulletin No. 104: antibiotic prophylaxis for gynecologic procedures. Obstet Gynecol. 2009;113(5):1180–9.
67. Agostini A, Cravello L, Shojai R, Ronda I, Roger V, Blanc B. Postoperative infection and surgical hysteroscopy. Fertil Steril. 2002;77(4):766–8.
68. Cooper NA, Smith P, Khan KS, Clark TJ. Vaginoscopic approach to outpatient hysteroscopy: a systematic review of the effect on pain. BJOG. 2010;117:532–9.
69. Sharma M, Taylor A, di Spiezio Sardo A, Buck L, Mastrogamvrakis G, Kosmas I, et al. Outpatient hysteroscopy: traditional versus the 'no-touch' technique. BJOG. 2005;112:963–7.
70. Clark TJ, Voit D, Song F, Hyde C, Gupta JK, Khan KS. Accuracy of hysteroscopy in the diagnosis of endometrial cancer and disease: a systematic review. JAMA. 2002;288:1610–21.
71. Cooper NA, Clark TJ, Middleton L, et al. Outpatient versus inpatient uterine polyp treatment for abnormal uterine bleeding: randomised controlled non-inferiority study. Br Med J. 2015;350:h1398.
72. Kremer C, Duffy S. A randomised controlled trial comparing transvaginal ultrasound, outpatient hysteroscopy and endometrial biopsy with inpatient hysteroscopy and curettage. BJOG. 2000;107:1058–9.
73. Litta P, Cosmi E, Saccardi C, Esposito C, Rui R, Ambrosini G. Outpatient operative polypectomy using a 5 mm hysteroscope without anaesthesia and/or analgesia: advantages and limits. Eur J Obstet Gynecol Reprod Biol. 2008;139(2):210–4.
74. Valle RF. Office hysteroscopy. Clin Obstet Gynecol. 1999;42:276–89.
75. Agostini A, Bretelle F, Cravello L, Maisonneuve AS, Roger V, Blanc B. Acceptance of outpatient flexible hysteroscopy by premenopausal and postmenopausal women. J Reprod Med. 2003;48:441–3.
76. Kremer C, Barik S, Duffy S. Flexible outpatient hysteroscopy without anaesthesia: a safe, successful and well tolerated procedure. Br J Obstet Gynaecol. 1998;105:672–6.
77. Chang CC. Efficacy of office diagnostic hysterofibroscopy. J Minim Invasive Gynecol. 2007;14:172–5.
78. Zlatkov V, Kostova P, Barzakov G, et al. Flexible hysteroscopy in irregular uterine bleeding. J BUON. 2007;12:53–6.
79. Salim S, et al. Diagnosis and management of endometrial polyps: a critical review of the literature. J Minim Invasive Gynecol. 2011;18(5):569–81.

80. Preutthipan S, Herabutya Y. Hysteroscopic polypectomy in 240 premenopausal and post-menopausal women. Fertil Steril. 2005;83:705–9.
81. Jansen FW, Vredevoogd CB, van Ulzen K, Hermans J, Trimbos JB, Trimbos-Kemper TC. Complications of hysteroscopy: a prospective, multicenter study. Obstet Gynecol. 2000;96(2):266–70.
82. Taskin O, Sadik S, Onoglu A, et al. Role of endometrial suppression on the frequency of intrauterine adhesions after resectoscopic surgery. J Am Assoc Gynecol Laparosc. 2000;7:351–4.
83. Emanuel MH, Wamsteker K. The Intra Uterine Morcellator: a new hysteroscopic operating technique to remove intrauterine polyps and myomas. J Minim Invas Gynecol. 2005;12(1):62–6.
84. Van Dongen H, Emanuel MH, Wolterbeek R, Trimbos JB, Jansen FW. Hysteroscopic morcellator for removal of intrauterine polyps and myomas: a randomized controlled pilot study among residents in training. The. J Minim Invasive Gynecol. 2008;15(4):466–71.
85. Vilos GA. Intrauterine surgery using a new coaxial bipolar electrode in normal saline solution (Versapoint): a pilot study. Fertil Steril. 1999;72:740–3.
86. Garuti G, Centinaio G, Luerti M. Outpatient hysteroscopic polypectomy in postmenopausal women: a comparison between mechanical and electrosurgical resection. J Minim Invasive Gynecol. 2008;15:595–600.
87. Timmermans A, Veersema S. Ambulatory transcervical resection of polyps with the Duckbill polyp snare: a modality for treatment of endometrial polyps. J Minim Invasive Gynecol. 2005;12:37–9.
88. Muzii L, Bellati F, Pernice M, Manci N, Angioli R, Panici PB. Resectoscopic versus bipolar electrode excision of endometrial polyps: a randomized study. Fertil Steril. 2007;87(4):909–17.
89. Smith PP, Middleton LJ, Connor M, Clark TJ. Hysteroscopic morcellation compared with electrical resection of endometrial polyps: a randomized controlled trial. Obstet Gynecol. 2014;123(4):745–51.
90. Orhue AA, Aziken ME, Igbefoh JO. A comparison of two adjunctive treatments for intrauterine adhesions following lysis. Int J Gynaecol Obstet. 2003;82(1):49–56.
91. Shveiky D, Rojansky N, Revel A, Benshushan A, Laufer N, Shushan A. Complications of hysteroscopic surgery: "Beyond the learning curve". J Minim Invasive Gynecol. 2007;14(2):218–22.
92. Technology assessment No. 7: Hysteroscopy. Obstet Gynecol. 2011;117(6):1486–91.
93. Schorge JO, Schaffer JI, Halvorson LM, Hoffman BL, Bradshaw KD, Cunningham FG. Williams gynecology. 1st ed. New York, NY: McGraw-Hill Medical; 2008.
94. Deans R, Abbott J. Review of intrauterine adhesions. J Minim Invasive Gynecol. 2010;17(5):555–69.
95. Bosteels J, Kasius J, Weyers S, Broekmans FJ, Mol BWJ, D'Hooghe TM. Hysteroscopy for treating subfertility associated with suspected major uterine cavity abnormalities. Cochrane Database Syst Rev. 2015;(2):CD009461.
96. Valle RF. Therapeutic hysteroscopy in infertility. Int J Fertil. 1984;29:143–8.
97. Kalampokas T, Tzanakaki D, Konidaris S, Iavazzo C, Kalampokas E, Gregoriou O. Endometrial polyps and their relationship in the pregnancy rates of patients undergoing intrauterine insemination. Clin Exp Obstet Gynecol. 2012;39(3):299–302.
98. Lass A, Williams G, Abusheikha N, Brinsden P. The effect of endometrial polyps on outcomes of in vitro fertilization (IVF) cycles. J Assist Reprod Genet. 1999;16(8):410–5.
99. Tiras B, Korucuoglu U, Polat M, Zeyneloglu HB, Saltik A, Yarali H. Management of endometrial polyps diagnosed before or during ICSI cycles. Reprod Biomed Online. 2012;24(1):123–8.
100. Check JH, Bostick-Smith CA, Choe JK, Amui J, Brasile D. Matched controlled study to evaluate the effect of endometrial polyps on pregnancy and implantation rates following in vitro fertilization-embryo transfer (IVF-ET). Clin Exp Obstet Gynecol. 2011;38(3):206–8.
101. Cenksoy P, Ficicioglu C, Yıldırım G, Yesiladali M. Hysteroscopic findings in women with recurrent IVF failures and the effect of correction of hysteroscopic findings on subsequent pregnancy rates. Arch Gynecol Obstet. 2013;287(2):357–60.
102. Eryilmaz OG, Gulerman C, Sarikaya E, Yesilyurt H, Karsli F, Cicek N. Appropriate interval between endometrial polyp resection and the proceeding IVF start. Arch Gynecol Obstet. 2012;285(6):1753–7.

Hysteroscopic Myomectomy

6

Shilpa Sharma and Shalu Gupta

6.1 Introduction

Uterine fibroids are the most common benign tumors of women in the reproductive age group. On the basis of postmortem studies, the prevalence rates are quoted to be varying from 20% to 50% [1]. The age group found to be most commonly presenting with myomas is the reproductive age group.

These are smooth muscle cell tumors of the uterus and have interweaving fibrous tissues that may contain collagen, fibronectin, and proteoglycan [2]. Pathogenesis of myomas is still not clear, but both estrogen and progesterone are found to have a major role in the proliferation of the tumor [3, 4]. Fibroids are rarely seen before menarche and generally start regressing once a woman attains menopause. As the myomas grow, they usually follow the path of least resistance, i.e., either they grow toward the abdominal cavity or toward the uterine cavity becoming subserous or submucous fibroids, respectively (5–10% of uterine fibroids) [5].

Although all uterine fibroids arise from myometrium, they are classified by their location in the uterus into three major clinical categories: subserosal, submucosal, and intramural. There can be single or multiple myomas in a uterus.

Subserous myomas needs surgical removal if the size is more than 7 cm in size they do not need surgical removal. Sometimes myomas smaller than 7 cm may cause symptoms due to their location, i.e., either they may cause bladder symptoms if present anteriorly or bowel discomfort if posteriorly located, and it may necessitate its removal. Myomectomy for subserous fibroids is either done laparoscopically or by a laparotomy. Similarly, **intramural fibroid** may be removed laparoscopically or by a laparotomy. Laparoscopic myomectomy has many advantages over laparotomy due to shorter convalescence period and better cosmesis. Laparoscopic myomectomy includes

S. Sharma, DGO, DNB, MNAMS, FNB (✉)
Aveya Natural IVF Fertility Centre, Delhi, India

S. Gupta, MS, DNB, MNAMS, FNB
IVF and Fertility, Cloud 9, Gurugram, Haryana, India

© Springer Nature Singapore Pte Ltd. 2018
S. Jain, D. B. Inamdar (eds.), *Manual of Fertility Enhancing Hysteroscopy*,
https://doi.org/10.1007/978-981-10-8028-9_6

removal of the myoma as well as repair of the myometrium through the endoscope; hence it requires more technical expertise than most other procedures which are done laparoscopically. The use of laparoscopic myomectomy is now gaining widespread acceptance due to increased training as well as availability of better equipment.

Women with **submucous fibroids** present with clinical symptoms such as menorrhagia, spasmodic dysmenorrhea, and inability to conceive in some. Submucous fibroids can arise from the anterior, posterior, or the lateral wall of the uterus. These are most commonly located at the body of the uterus but may also be present at the fundus or the isthmus. If present at the cornual end, then it may cause infertility by interfering with the transfer of the sperm at the uterotubal junction [6]. These myomas are found to have higher rate of malignant transformation and increased association with chronic endometritis [6]. Incidence of antenatal and postnatal complications such as preterm labor, postpartum hemorrhage, and operative deliveries is higher in women with submucous fibroid [7].

Submucous myomas can be treated by hysteroscopic resection or by subtotal or total hysterectomy through open or laparoscopic access. Hysteroscopic techniques are now preferred as it preserves fertility, is less invasive, and retains the menstural functions in the women, too. However some myomas may not be amenable to be treated hysteroscopically.

6.2 History of Hysteroscopic Myomectomy

Initially fibroids were treated with either by performing hysterectomy or doing a myomectomy through laparotomy. But with the developments in surgical techniques and instrumentation, accessibility of fibroids became easy with the application of laparoscopy. As the hysteroscope was introduced, the submucous fibroids became accessible and could be removed from the inner surface of the uterus. Initially the myomas were removed either by twisting the pedicles of the pedunculated fibroids with the help of ovum forceps or the fibroid pedicle would be cut with the help of scissors inserted through the hysteroscopic sheath.

In 1976, Neuwirth and Amin first reported resection of a fibroid using a resectoscope used in urology. They had used 32% dextran as a distension medium and monopolar current [8]. Later in 1987, Hallez used a specially designed resectoscope that used 1.5% glycine with continuous flow and cutting current [9].

With advances in instruments and increase in knowledge, hysteroscopic myomectomy is now the standard technique for management of submucous myomas.

6.3 Presurgical Evaluation of Submucous Fibroids

Removal of submucous myoma can be difficult most of the times, and hence it is necessary to decide the extent of the myoma before attempting the procedure. Fibroids can be evaluated using either transvaginal ultrasound scanning

(TVS) and/or sonohysterography (SHG) and office hysteroscopy. These diagnostic modalities enable us to assess the location, number, and size of the fibroid and also the depth of myometrial extension. SHG or office hysteroscopy delineates the intracavitary component of the fibroid as well as it may show any other intracavitary pathology. In a comparative study published in 2011, saline infusion sonography had a sensitivity of 99% and positive predictive value of 96% for submucous myomas. Hysteroscopy had a sensitivity, specificity, positive predictive value, and negative predictive value of 98%, 83%, 96%, and 91%, respectively, for all pathologies of the uterus. In conclusion, SIS was found to be superior to the TVS for diagnosing uterine pathologies and is equivalent to hysteroscopy, which is considered as the gold standard [10].

SHG is superior to TVS as it identifies not only the exact location of fibroid but also the exact proportion of the myoma that protrudes into the uterine cavity and hence helps in classifying the myoma and also deciding on the mode of treatment. In cases of multiple fibroids, or if differentiation between adenomyosis and fibroid is difficult or in obese patients where TVS or SIS is technically difficult to perform, magnetic resonance imaging (MRI) may be helpful [11, 12].

6.4   Classification of Submucous Fibroids

The classification used most commonly was developed in 1993 by Wamsteker et al. and adopted by the European Society for Gynecological Endoscopy (ESGE). This classification only considers the degree of myometrial penetration of the submucous fibroid (Table 6.1) [13].

In 2005, Lasmar et al. proposed a new classification of submucous fibroids that can be used preoperatively. This system of classification considers the degree of penetration of fibroid into the myometrium, extension of the base of the fibroid in relation to the wall of the uterus, size of the fibroid (in cm), and location of fibroid (Table 6.2). For each parameter, a score is given ranging from 0 to 2, and depending on the total score, patients are divided into three groups. The Lasmar score is found to have a better correlation to the surgical outcome as compared to when only the ESGE classification was used [14, 15].

Table 6.1 ESGE classification of submucous myomas [13]

Type 0	Entirely within the endometrial cavity
	No myometrial extension (pedunculated)
Type I	<50% myometrial extension
	<90° angle of myoma surface to uterine wall
Type II	≥50% myometrial extension
	≥90° angle of myoma surface to uterine wall

Table 6.2 Step W classification of submucous myomas [14]

	Size (cm)	Topography	Extension of the base	Penetration	Lateral wall	Total
0	<2	Low	<1/3	0		
1	2–5	Middle	1/3–2/3	<50%		
2	>5	Upper	>2/3	>50%	+1	
Score	**Group**	**Complexity and therapeutic options**				
0–4	I	Low complexity hysteroscopic myomectomy				
5–6	II	High complexity hysteroscopic myomectomy. Consider GnRH use. Consider two-step hysteroscopic technique				
7–9	III	Consider alternatives to hysteroscopic technique				

Source: Lasmar RB et al. Submucous myomas: a new presurgical classification to evaluate the viability of hysteroscopic surgical treatment—preliminary report. J Minimal Invasive Gynecol, 2005; 12(4):308–11. Reproduced with permission from Ricardo Lasmar

6.5   Instruments

Operative hysteroscope or resectoscope is the main equipment required for removal of submucous myoma. It has channels for instillation of medium, for the telescope and an extra channel for the insertion of operative devices such as loops or electrodes. Both monopolar as well as bipolar electrosurgical equipment can be used, though the distension media would change as discussed in the chapter of instruments. The use of monopolar currents requires a nonconducting media such as sorbitol 5% or glycine. The use of bipolar current has been found to be much safer and hence now preferred by most surgeons.

6.6   Hysteroscopic Techniques

The surgical technique would mainly depend upon the type of the myoma and its location in the endometrial cavity. Also the experience or the expertise of the surgeon may favor one technique over the other [16].

6.6.1   Office Hysteroscopic Myomectomy

Advent of smaller diameter hysteroscopes of diameters of 3–5 mm has now allowed many uterine pathologies to be treated without the need of cervical dilation and anesthesia and hence tackled at outpatient department itself. Smaller fibroids that are completely within the uterine cavity (G0) can be treated in office settings. The fibroid is first divided into two halves, and then each half is separated from the base in two or three slicing attempts. These are then pulled out with the help of a grasper.

Evidence is limited due to methodological weaknesses of studies evaluating hysteroscopic myomectomy in office settings, such as absence of a control group and short follow-up period. Larger trials are required to further evaluate the usefulness of this technique.

6.6.2   Fibroids Completely Within the Uterine Cavity (G0)

6.6.2.1 Resectoscopic Excision by Slicing

The method of slicing consists of repeated and progressive passage of the cutting loop through the fibroid starting from the top and then proceeding downward to the base. This procedure is also useful for the pedunculated fibroids (Figs. 6.1, 6.2, 6.3, 6.4, and 6.5).

During the resection of the fibroid, the fragments of the fibroids start accumulating within the cavity making the visibility poor, and these may require removal before any further attempt to slice and complete the procedure. The best way to remove them is under direct vision after grasping the loose tissue with loop or grasping forceps. Nowadays resectoscope with automatic chip aspiration is also available. The procedure should be considered complete when

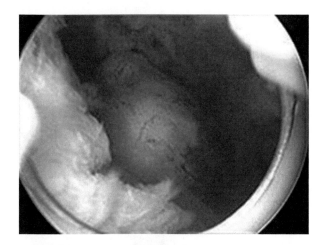

Fig. 6.1 Hysteroscopic view of submucous myoma before myomectomy

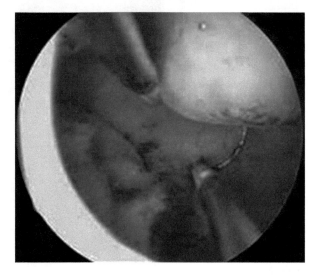

Fig. 6.2 Removal of myoma with slicing technique with the help of a cutting loop

Fig. 6.3 Partially removed
myoma

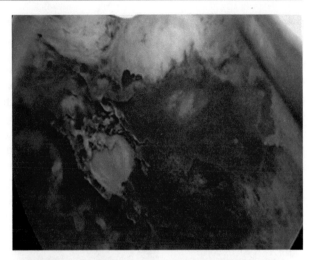

Fig. 6.4 Completely
removed myoma

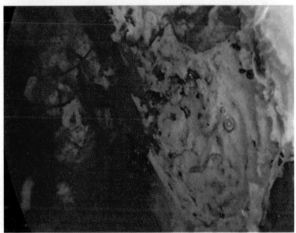

Fig. 6.5 Panoramic view
of the cavity after removal
of myoma

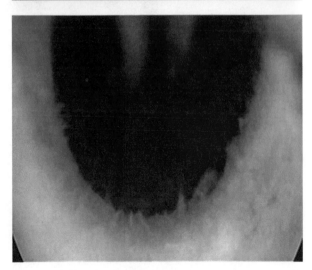

the base is smooth and regular and the fasciculate structure of the myometrium can be seen.

6.6.2.2 Cutting the Base of the Fibroid and then Extracting the Fibroid

In case of a pedunculated fibroid, the pedicle may be cut with the help of either a loop electrode or Nd: YAG laser. The fibroid can then be removed either under direct vision using Issaacson optical tenaculum or blindly using forceps. Some surgeons leave the resected fibroid tissue inside the cavity itself so that it is extruded during menstruation later.

6.6.2.3 Ablation by Nd: YAG laser

Small fibroids (<2 cm) can be ablated using Nd: YAG laser. In this method, the laser is first used to ablate the superficial blood vessels followed by dragging the laser against the fibroid multiple times, till the entire tissue is flattened out. This is known as the *touch technique*. The disadvantage of the technique is that no tissue is available for histopathology and also that the laser equipment is expensive and hence limiting its use.

6.6.2.4 Vaporization of Fibroid

In this technique spherical or cylindrical electrodes are used for vaporization of the fibroid. The electrode is moved slowly over the fibroid, and the current is only applied when we are moving toward the surgeon. This technique is continued till the myoma is reduced to such a size that can be easily removed by a tenaculum or a forceps.

The disadvantages of this technique are uterine perforation, gas embolism, and unavailability of tissue for histopathology. These complications can be managed by taking certain precautions during surgery. The surgeon should take care of the time for which the pressure has been applied, wattage of current used. The anesthetist should constantly monitor the end-tidal CO_2 of the patient and keep the operator informed avoiding serious complications.

6.6.2.5 Morcellation by Intrauterine Morcellator (IUM)

A newer technique that is morcellation by IUM preserves tissue for histological examination. This technique is effective for fibroids that are classified as G0 and G1 but not for G2. This technique may have a shorter learning curve and is faster as the tissue fragments are aspirated through the instrument only. This is a newer technique; hence further studies are needed for long-term follow-up and complications.

A retrospective comparative study was conducted in two centers from January 2012 to December 2013 with a total of 83 patients with submucous myomas type 0, 1, and 2. Thirty-four patients underwent hysteroscopic morcellation using MyoSure, and 49 had hysteroscopic resection using Versapoint-24F bipolar loop. There were 36 (71%) type 0 and 1 myomas and 15 (29%) type 2 in morcellation group versus

44 (59%) myomas type 0 and 1 and 31 (41%) type 2 in electrosurgical resection group ($p = 0.17$). The mean operative duration was 30 min in morcellation group, compared to 31 min in bipolar resection group ($p = 0.98$). Complete myoma removal was achieved in 22 (64%) patients in morcellation group and in 34 (69%) in bipolar resection group ($p = 0.65$). There were no differences in the adverse events between both groups. The prevalence of postoperative intrauterine adhesion was 10% in morcellation group and 13.8% in bipolar resection group ($p = 0.69$). In this short comparative series, hysteroscopic morcellation and bipolar loop resection were associated with comparable results for removal of submucous myomas [17].

6.6.3   Fibroids with Intramural Component (G1–G2)

Fibroids with intramural component are best treated in hands of experts as these are technically challenging with higher chances of complications. Fibroids with size more than 5 cm and with intramural components, i.e., G1 or G2, should not be removed hysteroscopically, as there are chances of incomplete resection and makes the surgery difficult.

Several techniques have been described having the same objective, i.e., to make intramural component as intracavitary.

6.6.3.1 Excision of the Intracavitary Component Only

Several authors in the past proposed that only the intracavitary portion of the fibroid could be excised leaving behind the intramural component [8]. It was on the assumption that the endometrium may grow over the intramural component and hence the fibroid may behave as an intramural one. But this proved to be useless because as the fibroid grew, it would have an intracavitary expulsion due to volumetric expansion, and hence the symptoms would persist. This procedure finally fell into disrepute.

6.6.3.2 Fibroid Excision Using the Two-Step Technique

This procedure was first described in 1990 by Donnez [18]. The procedure is based on the fact that as the myomectomy of intracavitary portion of myoma is performed, the intramural component grows toward the uterine cavity becoming intracavitary. In his first published paper in 1990, he treated 12 patients using this technique. Later on he published another study which had 78 patients in whom the largest portion of the myoma was present in the myometrium. In these set of patients, only four patients needed a third operative hysteroscopy, whereas 95% of patients only needed two hysteroscopies [19].

Steps of this technique:

1. The patient receives 8 weeks of GnRH agonist prior to scheduled surgery.
2. First hysteroscopy: Removal of the intracavitary portion of myoma using the splicing technique. After this the laser is made to enter the myoma at 90° angle, and the myolysis is done to shrink the size of the myoma. This is the first surgical step.

3. The patient now receives 8 weeks of GnRH agonist.
4. Second look hysteroscopy is performed, and the residual intracavitary fibroid is removed by the splicing technique.

The advantage of this procedure is that it is safe as it involves the removal of intracavitary portion only. But the disadvantages are that it involves two separate interventions. This may as well increase the cost of the procedure due to two surgeries involved as well as the need of multiple GnRH agonist injection. Only myomas with a reduced intramural development or of small dimensions can be treated with this technique.

6.6.3.3 One-Step Techniques for Complete Excision of Myoma

1. **Excision of intramural component by slicing**
   After the removal of the intracavitary portion by the splicing technique, the intramural portion is also removed in the similar manner. During the procedure the infusion of the media is stopped and restarted intermittently which leads to start of uterine contractions and changes the intrauterine pressure causing uterine massage which pushes the myoma into the cavity from the intramural region. This step is continued several times along with manual uterine massage till the entire tissue has been extruded and removed.

   In a study published by Zayed et al. which included 49 patients, the mean diameter of the myoma removed was 51.94 ± 5.58 mm. Complete resection of myoma by this technique was possible in 45 (91.84%) of women. Out of the 17 women who had infertility, 9 did conceive. One-step complete resection of myoma was more successful if myoma was single (97.5%), the size was <6 cm (97.73%), or Lasmar score was <7 (100%) [20].

   The complications associated with this technique are bleeding, intravasation, and perforation. The use of electrosurgical current while working at the intramural portion of myoma may also damage the adjacent normal myometrium.

2. **"Cold loop" myomectomy**
   In 1995 Mazzon first described this technique using cold loop, and it involves three steps [21]:
   (a) **Excision of the intracavitary component**: The intracavitary portion of the myoma is removed using the splicing technique. The excision stops at the level of the endometrial surface. This helps during the next step to identify the cleavage plane between the myoma and the myometrium.
   (b) **Enucleation of the intramural component**: Now the cold loop is inserted at the edge of the myoma at the endo-myometrial interface, and the fibroid is dissected away from the myometrium. During this step no electrosurgical current is used, and the loop is used mechanically or in cold manner. Subsequently a single tooth loop is used to hook out and also cut the fibrous bridges between the myoma and the myometrium.
   (c) **Excision of the intramural component**: Once the fibroid has been enucleated, the myoma now lies within the cavity, and this is further treated as intracavitary fibroid.

The disadvantages of this procedure are that it needs an experienced surgeon and the availability of a cold loop that limits its use. Studies to assess its efficacy are still lacking.

3. **In toto enucleation**
   (a) **Litta's technique**: With the Collin's knife, an elliptical incision is made at the endometrium at the interface of the myoma and the uterus till the zone where the cleavage between the myoma and the myometrium can be started. Connecting fibrous tissues are cut, the myoma is pushed into the cavity, and the myoma is then removed using the splicing technique. This technique was used successfully in 41 patients out of total of 44 patients with submucous fibroids (G2) with mean size of 3.2 cm (range 2–4 cm) [22].
   (b) **Lasmar's technique**: This technique was successfully used in 98 women where an "L"-shaped Collins electrode was used to cut the endometrium around the myoma, then mobilizing the fibroid from all directions into the cavity. Once the myoma is intracavitary, then it was either removed by splicing or in cases of small fibroids with the help of the grasper [14].
4. **Two resectoscope techniques** have been described but is limited in its use due to feasibility of the procedure [23]. This technique uses two resectoscopes of 7 and 9 mm size and hence its name. First using the smaller diameter resectoscope, the myoma is cut deep enough till the top of the myoma with an irregular surface is visualized, which is easier to grasp. The myoma is further dissected, and a specially designed myoma grasper further pulls the myoma into the cavity, using rotating and pulling action that completes the procedure. In case of inability to remove due to larger size of myoma, 9 mm resectoscope can be used to remove part of myoma to make passage smooth.

6.7 Outcomes of Hysteroscopic Myomectomy

Hysteroscopic myomectomy is proved by most studies to be both effective and a safe technique for treating menstrual disorders with up to 70–99% efficacy [24]. A number of factors may affect the success rate such as incomplete removal of the myoma and other causes of menorrhagia as well as development of a new fibroid. The size and number of fibroid have value in prognosticating the patient before the surgery. The surgical technique of myomectomy does not affect the success rates [25]. Various studies have evaluated the effect of hysteroscopic myomectomy on the reproductive outcome of the infertile women [26–29, 31]. The pregnancy rates reported after the hysteroscopic myomectomy varies from 16.7% to 76.9% with a mean of 45%. Such a disparity in the reported success rates is likely due to some other associated factor for infertility, discrepancy in follow-up, or differences in characteristics of patients including age and whether they had primary or secondary infertility [27]. As widely investigated, myomas as a sole cause of infertility is very uncommon and is thought to be sole cause in 1% of women; therefore, reproductive outcome after hysteroscopic myomectomy is influenced by other factors as well.

Fernandez et al. in 2001 reported that if fibroid was the sole cause of infertility, then pregnancy rate of 41.6% can be achieved by its removal; if one or more factors were present, the pregnancy rates were 26.3% and 6.3%, respectively [28].

Previously infertile women with G0 and G1 class of fibroids are likely to be benefitted from hysteroscopic myomectomy [29]. This was in contrast to women with G2 fibroids who did not show any benefit in comparison to the control group (women who had not undergone hysteroscopic myomectomy).

Many meta-analyses have assessed the impact of fibroids on IVF cycles [26, 27, 29].

Pritts compared infertile women with and without submucosal fibroids and found a significantly lower pregnancy rate (RR 0.32), implantation rate (RR 0.28), and delivery rates (RR 0.75) in patients with submucosal fibroids [26]. An updated meta-analysis by Somigliana et al. also found a significantly lower pregnancy and delivery rates for women with submucosal fibroids [odds ratio (OR), 0.3] [27]. Even Donnez and Jadoul found that submucous myomas are associated with lower pregnancy rates [29].

Only two studies evaluated IVF outcome after hysteroscopic myomectomy [32, 33]. Meta-analysis of these two retrospective studies reports that hysteroscopic myomectomy does not negatively affect the chances of pregnancy in IVF cycles [27]. However these results have to be taken with caution as they are on basis of two retrospective studies with few patients only.

6.8 Operative and Long-Term Complications

Hysteroscopic myomectomy as compared to other hysteroscopic procedures is associated with higher incidence of complications. Complication rate is reported to be between 0.3% and 28%. The two most frequent complications are fluid overload and uterine perforation. Other complications include cervical injury, air embolism, and bleeding. Late sequel includes intrauterine adhesions (IUA) and uterine rupture during subsequent pregnancy [34].

6.8.1 Uterine Perforation

Perforation of the uterus may occur during dilatation of the cervix while inserting the hysteroscope or during resection of myoma. The chances of perforation are increased if there is a large intramural component or an aggressive resection is carried out for the intramural portion [35]. The management of perforation would depend on the condition of the patient as well as whether any surrounding structure has been damaged or not.

In a study published in year 2003, data was collected from five hospitals over a period of 12 years. Overall 3541 hysteroscopic electrosurgeries were performed, of which 1468 cases were of transcervical resections of endometrium (TCRE), 797 cases of transcervical resection of myoma (TCRM), 783 cases of transcervical resection of endometrial polyp (TCRP), 189 cases of transcervical resection of uterine septa (TCRS), 112 cases of transcervical resection of uterine adhesion (TCRA), and 192 cases of transcervical removal of foreign body (TCRF). All surgeries were performed under ultrasonographic or laparoscopic guidance. Cases of uterine perforation were divided into two groups: entry-related or technique-related.

Uterine perforation was observed in 16 cases (0.45%). Out of these 16 cases, seven were due to cervical dilatation, one was due to insertion of the hysteroscope, and eight were caused by electrode. The incidences of uterine perforation of different operations were TCRA 4.46% (5/112), TCRF 3.12% (6/192), TCRE 0.27% (4/1468), TCRM 0.13% (1/797), and TCRP and TCRS none. These 16 cases were all diagnosed during operations, ten cases (62%) by 2D ultrasound and (or) laparoscopy and six cases (38%) by hysteroscopy and clinical features. 13 cases were complete uterine perforations, among them two were diagnosed by laparoscopic monitoring, five by ultrasound monitoring, four by hysteroscopy, and two by symptoms and ultrasound, and three cases were incomplete uterine perforations in which two were diagnosed by laparoscopic monitoring and one by ultrasound monitoring. According to the authors as the half of uterine perforation cases happened while entering into the uterine cavity, hence utmost attention is needed while introducing dilator or hysteroscope. The other half was related to technique, and hence the type of surgery and surgeons experience is of importance [36].

6.8.2   Intravasation and Electrolyte Imbalance

This has been categorized as the most serious complication of hysteroscopic myomectomy. At present a standard definition of fluid overload is lacking. The intravasation of the fluid used to distend the uterine cavity can cause hyponatremia, pulmonary/cerebral edema, heart failure, and even death [35, 37]. The fluid is absorbed mainly via the vessels in the myoma and also through peritoneal absorption. Fluid deficit of 1000 mL of nonelectrolyte media causes drop of serum sodium of 10 nmol/L, making 1000 mL as cutoff for nonelectrolyte media. With isotonic electrolyte media used with bipolar systems, deficit of even >1000 mL can be easily tolerated by healthy women, but the same may not be true with advanced age and with associated comorbidities (weight/cardiovascular or renal diseases, etc.). So the upper safe limit for isotonic media still remains undefined especially in relation to age, weight, and medical fitness of woman [38].

The main factor responsible for extravasation seems to be the intramural extension of the fibroid mainly due to damage to larger-sized vessels. Other factors include being the length of the operation, the size of the fibroid, and the total inflow volume. Till the evidence to define an upper safe threshold for isotonic media is absent, the BSGE/ESGE Guideline Development Group recommends a limit of 2500 mL for healthy fit women [38]. However, in the elderly or those with comorbid conditions such as cardiovascular disease and renal disorders, the thresholds should be lowered, and upper limits for fluid deficits should be 750 mL for hypotonic solutions and 1500 mL for isotonic solutions [38].

During surgery a close watch on the fluid balance, difference in the amount of inflow and outflow including the fluid that has leaked through the vagina, should be noted. The procedure should be abandoned before excessive fluid is absorbed. The use of bipolar instruments along with normal saline has reduced this complication tremendously.

6.8.3 Postoperative Intrauterine Adhesions

The incidence of postoperative IUA after hysterosocpic myomectomy ranges from 1% to 13% [39]. One can minimize the risk by avoiding forceful manipulation and trauma to healthy tissue around the fibroid. Surgeon should use minimal electrosurgery during the surgery especially in cases with multiple fibroids. One can use either barrier agents such as levonorgestrel-releasing intrauterine device or Foley's catheter to reduce the development of adhesions. Postoperative use of estrogens and progesterones is also recommended by some authors. No single method has been proven to be efficacious at preventing the development of intrauterine adhesions following hysteroscopic operative procedures.

6.8.4 Uterine Rupture During Pregnancy

Uterine rupture may occur during future pregnancy especially if the myometrium has been disrupted during myomectomy. The patient should be explained about the risk of uterine rupture and advised to avoid pregnancy for at least a year. Although only very few cases of uterine perforation are reported [39–41], some surgeons prefer cesarean section over vaginal delivery in post myomectomy pregnancies. However, the evidence in support of cesarean section preventing uterine rupture is lacking.

Conclusions

Hysteroscopic removal of submucous myomas using the splicing technique is the most common and well-accepted technique for G0/G1 class of myomas. Among various other methods of hysteroscopic myomectomy, recently available intrauterine morcellator may be a valid alternative to the splicing method. Small fibroids can be treated at outpatient department with the use of small diameter office hysteroscopes. Various techniques for complete removal of the myoma have been described that may include the use of hydro-dissection, GnRH agonist, and even the two-stage surgical technique, but mostly these procedures have either limited success or very few studies to its credit hence limiting their widespread acceptance. Hence, the surgical management of G2 submucous myoma needs greater technical expertise because not only it is technically difficult but is also associated with higher complication rates. Careful selection of cases with thorough presurgical evaluation along with experienced surgeons in a fully equipped setup is recommended for hysteroscopic myomectomy.

References

1. Novak ER, Woodruff JD. Myoma and other benign tumors of the uterus. In:Gynecologic and obstetric pathology. 8th ed. Philadelphia, PA: W.B. Saunders; 1979. p. 260–78.
2. Parker WH. Etiology, symptomatology, and diagnosis of uterine myomas. Fertil Steril. 2007;87(4):725–36.
3. Rein MS, Barbieri RL, Friedman AJ. Progesterone: a critical role in the pathogenesis of uterine myomas. Am J Obstet Gynecol. 1995;172(1:14–8.
4. Andersen J. Growth factors and cytokines in uterine leiomyomas. Semin Reprod Endocrinol. 1996;14(3):269–82.
5. Ubaldi F, Tournaye H, Camus M, Van der Pas H, Gepts E, Devroey P. Fertility after hysteroscopic omy. Hum Reprod Update. 1995;1:81–90.
6. Valle RF, Baggish MS. Hysteroscopic myomectomy. In: Baggish MS, Valle RF, Guedj H, editors. Hysteroscopy. Visual perspectives of uterine anatomy, Physiology and pathology. Diagnostic and operative hysteroscopy. 3rd ed. Philadelphia, PA: Lippincott Williams & Wilkins, a Wolters Kluwer business; 2007. p. 385–404.
7. Bernard G, Darai E, Poncelet C, Benifla JL, Madelenat P. Fertility after hysteroscopic myomectomy: effect of intramural fibroids associated. Eur J Obstet Gynecol Reprod Biol. 2000;88:85–90.
8. Neuwirth RS, Amin HK. Excision of submucous fibroids with hysteroscopic control. Am J Obstet Gynecol. 1976;126:95–9.
9. Hallez JP. Single-stage total hysteroscopic myomectomies: indications, techniques, and results. Fertil Steril. 1995;63:703–8.
10. Bingol B, Gunenc Z, Gedikbasi A, Guner H, Tasdemir S, Tiras B. Comparison of diagnostic accuracy of saline infusion sonohysterography, transvaginal sonography and hysteroscopy. J Obstet Gynaecol. 2011;31(1):54–8.
11. Ahmed S, Zikri B, Aluwee S, Kato H, Zhou X, Hara T, Fujita H, et al. Magnetic resonance imaging of uterine fibroids: a preliminary investigation into the usefulness of 3D-rendered images for surgical planning. Springerplus. 2015;4:384.
12. Murase E, Siegelman ES, Outwater EK, Perez-Jaffe LA, Tureck RW. Uterine leiomyomas: histopathologic features, MR imaging findings, differential diagnosis, and treatment. Radiographics. 1999;19(5):1179–97.
13. Wamsteker K, Emanuel MH, de Kruif JH. Transcervical hysteroscopic resection of submucous fibroids for abnormal uterine bleeding: results regarding the degree of intramural extension. Obstet Gynecol. 1993;82(5):736–40.
14. Lasmar RB, Barrozo PR, Dias R, Oliveira MA. Submucous myomas: a new presurgical classification to evaluate the viability of hysteroscopic surgical treatment--preliminary report. J Minim Invasive Gynecol. 2005;12(4):308–11.
15. Lasmar RB, et al. A new system to classify submucous myomas: a Brazilian multicentre study. J Minim Invasive Gynecol. 2012;19(5):575–90.
16. Di Spiezio Sardo A, Mazzon I, Bramante S, Bettocchi S, Bifulco G, Guida M, Nappi C. Hysteroscopic myomectomy: a comprehensive review of surgical techniques. Hum Reprod Update. 2008;14(2):101–19.
17. Hamidouche A, Vincienne M, Thubert T, Trichot C, Demoulin G, Nazac A, Fernandez H, Rivain AL, Deffieux X. Operative hysteroscopy for myoma removal: morcellation versus bipolar loop resection. J Gynecol Obstet Biol Reprod. 2015;44(7):658–64. https://doi.org/10.1016/j.jgyn.2014.09.006. French
18. Donnez J, Nisolle M. Hysteroscopic surgery. Curr Opin Obstet Gynecol. 1992;4(3):439-46.
19. Donnez J, Polet R, Smets M, Bassil S, Nisolle M. Hysteroscopic myomectomy. Curr Opin Obstet Gynecol. 1995;7:311–16.
20. Zayed M, Fouda UM, Zayed SM, Elsetohy KA, Hashem AT. Hysteroscopic myomectomy of large submucous myomas in a 1-step procedure using multiple slicing sessions technique. J Minim Invasive Gynecol. 2015;22(7):1196–202.

21. Mazzon I, Favilli A, Grasso M, Horvath S, Di Renzo GC, Gerli S. Is cold loop hysteroscopic myomectomy a safe and effective technique for the treatment of submucous myomas with intramural development? A series of 1434 surgical procedures. J Minim Invasive Gynecol. 2015;22(5):792–8.
22. Litta P, Vasile C, Merlin F, Pozzan C, Sacco G, Gravila P, Stelia C. A new technique of hysteroscopic myomectomy with enucleation in toto. J Am Assoc Gynecol Laparosc. 2003;10:263–70.
23. Lin B, Akiba Y, Iwata Y. One-step hysteroscopic removal of sinking submucous fibroid in two infertile patients. Fertil Steril. 2000;74:1035–8.
24. Capmas P, Levaillant JM, Fernandez H. Surgical techniques and outcome in the management of submucous fibroids. Curr Opin Obstet Gynecol. 2013;25(4):332–8.
25. Emanuel MH, Wamsteker K, Hart AA, Metz G, Lammes FB. Long-term results of hysteroscopic myomectomy for abnormal uterine bleeding. Obstet Gynecol. 1999;93(5):743–8.
26. Pritts EA. Fibroids and infertility: a systematic review of the evidence. Obstet Gynecol Surv. 2001;56(8):483–91.
27. Somigliana E, Vercellini P, Daguati R, Pasin R, De Giorgi O, Crosignani PG. Fibroids and female reproduction: a critical analysis of the evidence. Hum Reprod Update. 2007;13(5):465–76.
28. Fernandez H, Sefrioui O, Virelizier C, Gervaise A, Gomel V, Frydman R. Hysteroscopic resection of submucosal myomas in patients with infertility. Hum Reprod. 2001;16(7):1489–92.
29. Donnez J, Jadoul P. What are the implications of myomas on fertility? A need for a debate? Hum Reprod. 2002;17(6):1424–30.
30. Shokeir TA. Hysteroscopic management in submucous fibroids to improve fertility. Arch Gynecol Obstet. 2005;273(1):50–4.
31. Surrey ES, Minjarez DA, Stevens JM, Schoolcraft WB. Effect of myomectomy on the outcome of assisted reproductive technologies. Fertil Steril. 2005;83:1473–9.
32. Narayan R, Rajat Goswamy K. Treatment of submucous fibroids, and outcome of assisted conception. J Am Assoc Gynecol Laparosc. 1994;1:307–11.
33. Paschopoulos M, Polyzos NP, Lavasidis LG, Vrekoussis T, Dalkalitsis N, Paraskevaidis E. Safety issues of hysteroscopic surgery. Ann N Y Acad Sci. 2006;1092:229–34.
34. Murakami T, Tamura M, Ozawa Y, Suzuki H, Terada Y, Okamura K. Safe techniques in surgery for hysteroscopic myomectomy. J Obstet Gynaecol Res. 2005;31:216–23.
35. Xia EL, Duan H, Zhang J, Chen F, Wang SM, Zhang PJ, Yu D, Zheng J, Huang XW. Analysis of 16 cases of uterine perforation during hysteroscopic electro-surgeries. Zhonghua Fu Chan Ke Za Zhi. 2003;38(5):280–3.
36. Pasini A, Belloni C. Intraoperative complications of 697 consecutive operative hysteroscopies. Minerva Ginecol. 2001;53(1):13–20.
37. AAGL, et al. AAGL Practice Report: practical Guidelines for the Management of hysteroscopic distension media. J Minim Invasive Gynecol. 2013;20:137–48.
38. Touboul C, Fernandez H, Deffieux X, Berry R, Frydman R, Gervaise A. Uterine synechiae after bipolar hysteroscopic resection of submucosal myomas in patients with infertility. Fertil Steril. 2009;92(5):1690–3.
39. Derman SG, Rehnstrom J, Neuwirth RS. The long-term effectiveness of hysteroscopic treatment of menorrhagia and leiofibroids. Obstet Gynecol. 1991;77:591–4.
40. Yaron Y, Shenhav M, Jaffa AJ, Lessing JB, Peyser MR. Uterine rupture at 33 weeks' gestation subsequent to hysteroscopic uterine perforation. Am J Obstet Gynecol. 1994;170(3):786–7.
41. Sentilhes L, Sergent F, Berthier A, Catala L, Descamps P, Marpeau L. Uterine rupture following operative hysteroscopy. Gynecol Obstet Fertil. 2006;34(11):1064–70.

Role of Hysteroscopy in Mullerian Anomalies

7

Jyoti Mishra

7.1 Introduction

Congenital uterine anomalies are developmental defects of Mullerian ducts during embryogenesis. These are categorized into defects of genesis and fusion.

References regarding the existence of Mullerian defects date back to antiquity, around 300 BC. Columbo reported the first documented case of vaginal agenesis (uterus and vagina) in the sixteenth century [1].

The exact incidence of congenital uterine anomalies is unknown because most women with such anomalies remain asymptomatic. Most of the studies measuring prevalence were conducted in a small population of women who have experienced a pregnancy loss; hence the actual prevalence in general population remains undetermined. Uterine anomalies occur in 2–4% of infertile women and fertile women with normal reproductive outcomes. The incidence is higher, however, among women with recurrent first-trimester miscarriage or late first- or second-trimester miscarriage/preterm delivery. Arcuate uterus, often diagnosed in women without any reproductive problems, is the most common uterine anomaly (5%), followed by septate uterus (3%) and bicornuate uterus (0.5%) [2].

Mullerian anomalies may present with a variety of gynecological and obstetrical problems [2, 3]. Uterine septum is the commonest uterine anomaly, responsible for approximately 80–90% of congenital uterine malformations [2]. Among all uterine malformations, uterine septum is the only one that can be treated and corrected by hysteroscopic surgery [3].

J. Mishra, MD (Obs & Gyn)
Jaypee Hospital, Noida, UP, India

© Springer Nature Singapore Pte Ltd. 2018
S. Jain, D. B. Inamdar (eds.), *Manual of Fertility Enhancing Hysteroscopy*,
https://doi.org/10.1007/978-981-10-8028-9_7

7.2   Etiology

The underlying etiology of congenital Mullerian defects is not well understood. The karyotype of women with these anomalies is usually normal. It is the process of embryogenesis that governs the malformations of the genital tract. The development of the uterus starts at around 8–16 weeks of fetal life from the paired paramesonephric (Mullerian) ducts. These ducts pass through three phases of development [4]:

- **Organogenesis**: Both paramesonephric ducts begin to develop.
- **Fusion**: Upper part of the vagina, cervix, and uterus are formed by lateral fusion of the lower Mullerian ducts. The upper cranial part of the Mullerian ducts remains unfused and forms the fallopian tubes.
- **Septal absorption**: Central septum left after the fusion of lower Mullerian ducts eventually gets absorbed after 9 weeks leading to single uterus and cervix.

A defect in the subperitoneal fibro-muscular tissue, which normally pulls the Mullerian duct together, an unusually thick round ligament or a tough vesicorectal fold, may contribute to developmental defects.

There is another set of ducts called mesonephric or Wolffian ducts which are crucial for renal development and also induce female reproductive tract development [5]. As a result, any abnormalities of mesonephric maldevelopment may also have an effect on genital tract formation [6]. Hence it is important to look for congenital abnormalities of renal system in patients where any genital anomaly is detected [7].

7.3   Classification

The most widely accepted classification of Mullerian duct anomalies is designed by American Fertility Society (AFS) (1988) (Table 7.1) [8]. Although this system is based on the clinically useful scheme of Buttram and Gibbons which combines the degree of developmental failure with clinical manifestations [9], it does not fully cover associated anomalies in the vagina, cervix, fallopian tubes, and renal system.

This system focuses largely on vertical fusion defects. Associated anomalies are not fully included, and a note of these should always be made. Detailed discussion of the classification would be beyond the prerogative of this chapter.

7.4   Signs and Symptoms

Complains suggestive of a uterine anomaly include dysmenorrhea, menstrual abnormalities (amenorrhea, hypomenorrhea), hematocolpos, recurrent miscarriage, malpresentation, and preterm delivery. The ability to achieve a clinical pregnancy is not typically impaired.

Table 7.1 AFS classification of Mullerian anomalies [8]

Class I	Hypoplasia and agenesis (a) vaginal (b) cervical (c) fundal (d) tubal (e) combined
Class II	Unicornuate • Communicating • Non-communicating • No cavity • No horn
Class III	Didelphys
Class IV	Bicornuate (a) partial (b) complete
Class V	Septate (a) partial (b) complete
Class VI	Arcuate
Class VII	DES drug related

A clinical examination may reveal a vaginal septum, double cervix, an unusually deviated uterus, or a very wide uterus to raise a suspicion of an anomaly.

7.5   Mullerian Anomalies and Reproductive Outcome

Different types of congenital uterine malformations may have different effects on reproductive performance [10]. Unicornuate uterus and uterus didelphys usually have a similar effect on pregnancy outcome [10–12]. Bicornuate and septate uterus both have incomplete absorption of septum as the etiological cause [11–14]. In patients with septate uteri, the reported incidence of abortion is 67%, prematurity 33%, and live births 28% [11].

Among various mechanisms proposed to explain the adverse effect of septate uterus on pregnancy outcome, the diminished size of uterine cavity and cervical incompetence have been suggested as the most probable etiological factors [13, 15]. Septum consisting of fibroelastic tissue with inadequate vascularization and having altered relations between myometrial and endometrial vessels can exert a negative effect on fetal placentation [12, 14, 16]. A contrasting study by Dabirashrafi et al. found significantly less connective tissue, a higher amount of muscle tissue, and more vessels in the septum. They suggested that pregnancy wastage is caused by poor decidualization and placentation. Reduced amounts of connective tissue and increased muscle content are said to cause uncoordinated contractility [15].

7.6   Diagnosis

For definitive diagnosis of Mullerian anomalies, one has to visualize both the internal and external uterine contour. Various diagnostic modalities have been utilized for uterine anomalies, each one having its own advantages and limitations. Two-dimensional ultrasonography or hysterosalpingography is an acceptable first-line screening tool.

7.6.1   Ultrasonography

Ultrasonography (USG) is useful for evaluating the kidneys, detecting hematometra or hematocolpos, and confirming the presence of ovaries in women with primary amenorrhea or diagnosis of septate uterus or agenesis. It also provides information about uterine contour, internal and external. In the secretory phase of the menstrual cycle, there is improved visualization of the endometrium. A 3D ultrasound can visualize the uterine cavity, myometrium, and the outer contour of the uterus in a single image, such as a coronal view. It is a noninvasive, reproducible, reliable method of differentiating the septate from the bicornuate uteri [16–18] (Fig. 7.1).

7.6.2   Hysterosalpingography

Hysterosalpingography (HSG) is a cost-effective modality of evaluating the uterine cavity for diagnosis of uterine anomalies. It is widely available even in low-cost settings. The advantage of hysterosalpingography is that it provides additional information of fallopian tube patency. The drawback of HSG is that it does not give any information of external uterine contour. To overcome this, additional modalities may be required for making a definitive diagnosis (Figs. 7.2 and 7.3).

7.6.3   Magnetic Resonance Imaging

Magnetic resonance imaging (MRI) can provide excellent delineation of internal as well as external contour of the uterus, without exposure to ionizing radiations. It

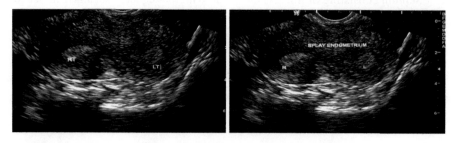

Fig. 7.1 (**a, b**) Ultrasound of bicornuate uterus (Courtesy Dr. Monika Kansal)

Fig. 7.2 HSG
bicornuate uterus

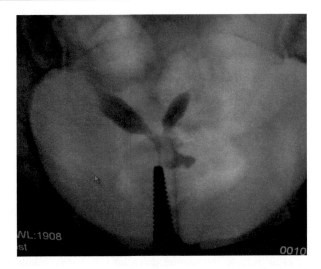

Fig. 7.3 Complete uterine
septum

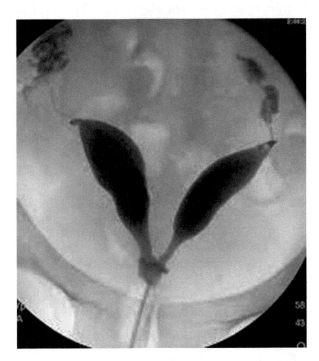

can also measure the intercornual diameter (>4 cm suggests a bicornuate/didelphys uterus and <2 cm suggests a septate uterus; measurements of 2–4 cm are indeterminate). MRI can distinguish between myometrial and fibrous septum of a bicornuate uterus and septate uterus, respectively. MRI can visualize the extent of the septum in both anomalies [19]. MR imaging may also be helpful in detecting a uterine horn and visualizing an endometrial stripe.

7.6.4   Hysteroscopy and Laparoscopy

Hysteroscopy enables direct visualization of the intrauterine cavity and ostia, hence very helpful in establishing correct diagnosis in suspected cases with abnormal HSG [20–22]. However, hysteroscopy has a limitation of inability to visualize the external contour of the uterus and is therefore often inadequate in differentiating between different types of malformations. Consequently, patients with a septum-like structure on HSG need a combined approach with diagnostic laparoscopy to differentiate bicornuate and septate uteri. In spite of newer technologies available, this combination (hysteroscopy/laparoscopy) is considered to be the gold standard in evaluating congenital uterine anomalies [20–23].

Hysteroscopy with laparoscopy offers the added advantage of concurrent treatment, as in the case of a uterine septum resection and other fertility enhancing surgery.

Hysteroscopy has the drawback of being an invasive procedure. With advancement in technology, smaller diameter telescopes, inbuilt cameras, and illumination systems, hysteroscopy nowadays is often performed under local anesthesia, in an office setting. Serious complications such as air embolism or uterine perforation can occur rarely [24].

7.7   Treatment

Most of the Mullerian anomalies are accidentally diagnosed during an infertility workup, during pregnancy or at childbirth. Restoration of normal uterine architecture and preservation of fertility are the goals of surgical treatment of uterine anomalies.

The commonest anomaly is a septate uterus. Surgical intervention for a septate uterus is needed only in patients with recurrent miscarriages. Infertility remains a controversial indication for performing septum resection.

7.8   Hysteroscopy in Mullerian Anomalies

Depending upon the degree of fusion defect, Mullerian anomalies can be classified as arcuate, partial, and complete septum.

7.8.1   Arcuate Uterus

Arcuate uterus is a condition in which the myometrium dips at the fundus and may form a small septation into the cavity. It is also defined as any fundal protrusion into the cavity that has an angle of more than 90°. The demarcation between an arcuate and a septate uterus remains undefined. Arcuate uterus is considered to be a normal variant in uterine shape, and most patients with an arcuate uterus do not require any

Fig. 7.4 Arcuate uterus

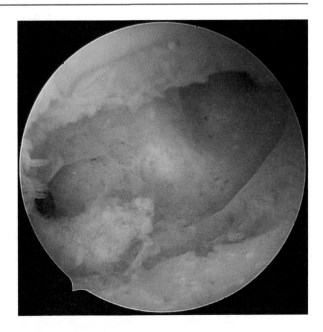

surgery. In patients with repeated pregnancy loss suspected to be due to an arcuate uterus, hysteroscopic resection can be considered, although there are no conclusive studies on the same (Fig. 7.4).

7.8.2 Uterine Septum

Uterine septum is the only Mullerian anomaly where hysteroscopy has a definite role in diagnosis and management. There is no doubt about the therapeutic effects of hysteroscopic metroplasty in patients with recurrent abortions and normal fertility. In patients with secondary infertility and recurrent spontaneous abortions, hysteroscopic metroplasty is applied as a treatment for their poor reproductive performance [25]. But the role of hysteroscopic septal resection as a prophylactic procedure is always debatable in patients presenting with primary unexplained infertility [14, 26].

Abdominal metroplasty by Jones and Tompkins technique for the incision of septum has been completely abandoned in favor of hysteroscopy, which has a much lower morbidity.

Timing of surgery: Best time to perform surgery is the postmenstrual or early follicular phase because the surrounding endometrium is thin and least vascular at this phase. Ostia which serve as important landmark are also clearly visible at this time.

Preoperative evaluation: Septal resection should be offered if there is history of poor reproductive performance rather than mere presence of a septate uterus [27]. Ideal candidates for surgery include women who had recurrent spontaneous abortions, a single second-trimester loss, or history of preterm delivery [28, 29].

Although few authors have tried pretreatment with gonadotropin-releasing hormone agonists to make the endometrium thin, there doesn't seem to be any definitive role in improving the surgical outcome.

Instrumentation: Hysteroscope 30°, 4 mm (widely available), and 2.9 mm (preferred for office procedures) (Figs. 7.5 and 7.6).

Distention medium: Normal saline can be used with bipolar instruments or when operative sheath and scissor are being used. It prevents complications of fluid overload. Glycine is required when monopolar current is being used.

Technique: Surgery begins with the insertion of a diagnostic hysteroscope, to confirm the diagnosis and to assess the extent and thickness of septum. This initial assessment helps in selection of the correct instrument and distension medium for the therapeutic procedure. Although it is preferred to use the narrowest sheath through vaginoscopy, one should not hesitate in dilating the cervix, if needed. Forceful entry through the cervix increases the risk of perforation or creation of a false passage. Serial dilatation with lubricated ends of dilators prevents this complication.

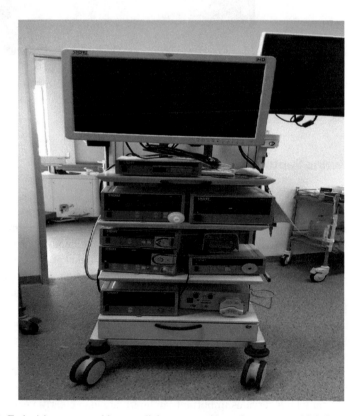

Fig. 7.5 Endovision system with xenon light source, camera, hysteromat with inflow and outflow tubes, and high-frequency, underwater electrosurgical unit

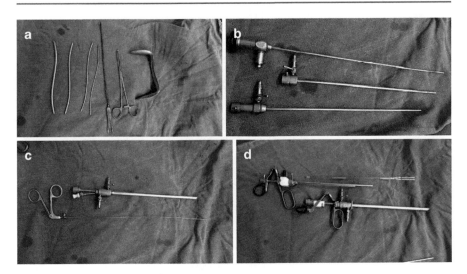

Fig. 7.6 (**a**) Minimum gynae instruments, (**b**) diagnostic sheath, (**c**) operative sheath and semi-rigid scissor, and (**d**) resectoscope, electrodes, and Collin's knife

Septum may be complete reaching up to the os and may have a cervical and vaginal component or partial (subseptate). It may have a broad or a narrow base at the fundus.

Combining laparoscopy is still considered to be the most accepted method to differentiate with bicornuate uterus. With advancements in technology, it is possible to confidently make a diagnosis of septum by a preoperative MRI or 3D scan. Hence in modern settings, laparoscopy may not be essential, just for confirmation of diagnosis of a bicornuate uterus.

A thin septum (<3 cm at fundus) can be easily cut with either a scissor through an operative sheath or Collin's knife through a resectoscope, starting from the most proximal (or caudal) end by straight incising movements. Once the fundus is approaching, the septum usually becomes broad. Here it is important to convert a broad septum into a narrow one, by incising the lateral sides first (Figs. 7.7, 7.8, and 7.9).

For a broad septum equal to or more than 3 cm at the fundus, the incision should begin at the lower most part, with scissors directed superiorly along the lateral margins of the septum, until it is incised up to 0.5 cm from its junction with the normal myometrium. The opposite lateral margin should be similarly incised.

This process is repeatedly performed alternatively on each side until the original V-shaped septum is reconfigured into a short, broad notch between the tubal ostia.

Fig. 7.7 Partial septum

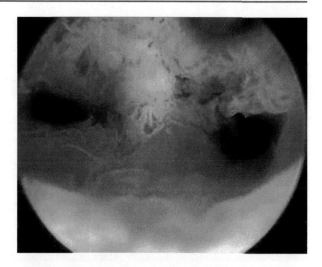

Fig. 7.8 Broad fundus with septum

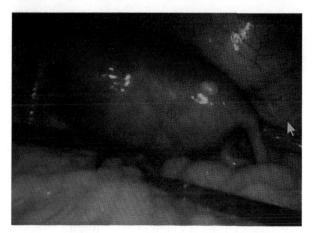

The notch is incised horizontally by a Collin's knife starting near one tubal ostium and progressing to the opposite side.

Usually the tendency of operator is to drift posteriorly during the dissection; hence it is important to consciously remain equidistant between the anterior and the posterior wall. Intermittent withdrawal of the hysteroscope to reorient in the cavity is an essential step to prevent perforation.

If two cervices are noted, a Foley balloon may be inserted into one os to prevent leakage of the distension media. Septum is incised at a point above the internal cervical os till the Foley's catheter is visualized. Uterine septum is then incised in the usual way. There is a controversy about increasing the risk of cervical incompetence, by cutting the cervical septum after unification of the cavity. There is a school of thought that it is better not to remove the cervical part in order to prevent cervical incompetence [30, 31]. Author does not support this hypothesis as also the work done by Donnez and Nisolle [32].

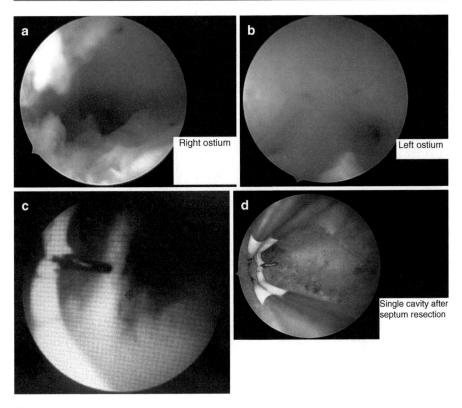

Fig. 7.9 Complete septum resection

It can be difficult to recognize the end point of septum dissection. One approach is to continue cutting until increased bleeding is noted, since the septum often has poor blood supply compared to the myometrium, but this approach will not work if a coagulative instrument is used.

If laparoscopy is performed at the same time, the laparoscope can be used to visualize when the hysteroscopic resection is getting too close to the uterine serosal surface, especially if the laparoscopic light is dimmed so that the hysteroscopic light can be appreciated.

On completion of the procedure, the surgeon should be able to visualize the fundus and sweep easily between ostia. The uterine cavity should appear normal.

7.9   Complications

7.9.1   Perforation

Three important landmarks in any hysteroscopic surgery are the internal os and the two ostia. Proper orientation by intermittent withdrawal of the hysteroscope up to the os and taking a panoramic view of the cavity help in preventing perforation.

The tendency to go too deep into the myometrium to complete the procedure needs to be discouraged. It is better to underdo the septum than overdoing it. Leaving behind a residual fundal notch up to 1 cm is accepted as a complete procedure.

7.9.2 Fluid Overload

General principles of quick surgery, maintaining input-output balance and using adequate pressure settings on hysteromat, prevent this complication. Although saline is safer than glycine, absorption of too much of any fluid should be avoided.

7.9.3 Residual Septa

Residual septa are a part of septa which persist post-surgery. Fedele L found incidence of residual septum of 44.1% in their study and concluded that the residual septum of <1 cm does not adversely affect on reproductive performance, and repeat surgery is therefore not indicated [33].

7.10 Postoperative Care

No further treatment is required postoperatively. Intrauterine devices, Foley balloons, high-dose estrogen, and antibiotics are not necessary [6]. Formation of intrauterine synechiae is rare, as are postoperative infections. Endogenous estrogen is sufficient to promote new endometrium within 2 months of hysteroscopic metroplasty [7]. In a randomized study by Dabirashrafi et al., there was no benefit of estrogen therapy after hysteroscopic metroplasty [33]. In spite of this, many surgeons still prefer to give conjugated estrogens 1.25 mg/day for 25 days and progesterone 10 mg/day added on days 21–25 after surgery to assist epithelialization.

An HSG should be performed 2 months after surgery to assess success. Typically, over 90% of the septum is removed during the procedure. Occasionally, further repairs of the septum are required, again in an ambulatory setting [6, 34]. In one series, a residual fundal notch >1 cm on follow-up hysteroscopy was considered as an indication for repeating septoplasty [35]. Attempts at pregnancy may begin 2 months postoperatively if the procedure is deemed adequate.

7.11 Outcome

There are not many randomized control trials on the outcome of surgery on reproductive outcome. One group reported a reduction in the rate of spontaneous abortions from 86% to 12% in 115 women [36]. Another study revealed an 86% delivery rate [37].

7.12   Hysteroscopy in Other Uterine Anomalies

Most of the Mullerian anomalies are diagnosed preoperatively by imaging. Sometimes in an unexpected case, if an anomaly is diagnosed during a hysteron-laparoscopy, one may use this modality to assess the size of the cavities. Didelphys and bicornuate uteri even though have a slightly smaller cavity, they do not need any surgical intervention.

Unicornuate uterus is a rare uterine malformation, with an incidence of 1 in 1,00,000. It is an outcome of incomplete development of one of the Mullerian ducts. Hence, a unicornuate uterus may not necessarily be associated with a rudimentary horn. Most of the rudimentary horns are non-communicating and are mostly connected with the uterus through a fibrous band.

The endometrium in the rudimentary horn may be functional or nonfunctional. Rarely an ectopic pregnancy may occur in the non-communicating rudimentary horn through transperitoneal migration of sperms or fertilized ovum from the contralateral tube. Unlike tubal ectopic pregnancy, which usually ruptures in first trimester, about 90% of these pregnancies culminate in rupture mostly in the second trimester. This is because the myometrium supporting and surrounding the gestational sac can expand with the growing fetus but only up to a certain extent. A functional rudimentary horn may develop endometriosis leading to severe menstrual pain. Treatment consists of excision of rudimentary horn (Figs. 7.10 and 7.11).

In a small study, hysteroscopic drainage of a hematometra in a functional non-communicating accessory horn of a unicornuate uterus was performed by using electrocautery to create a communication between the horns. At 1 month follow-up, a single uterine cavity was identified, and the symptoms were completely relieved. Further studies are required before these treatment modalities are widely accepted.

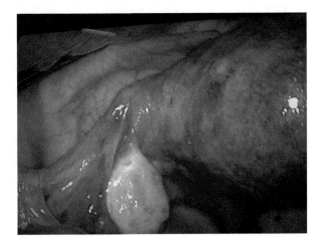

Fig. 7.10 Unicornuate uterus with a nonfunctional rudimentary horn

Fig. 7.11 Unicornuate
uterus with a hematometra
in non-communicating
horn with functional
endometrium

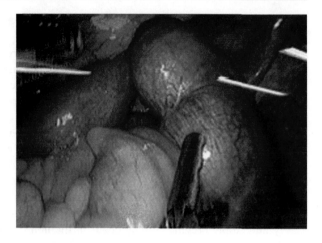

Conclusion

Mullerian anomalies are a diverse group of developmental defects of the female genital tract. Establishing an accurate diagnosis is essential to decide if any surgical intervention is required. Further management strategies will depend upon the patient's symptoms and the type of malformation. Ultimate goal of treatment is to achieve an anatomically and physiologically normal genital tract to fulfill healthy sexual relations and to achieve successful reproductive outcomes for the patient.

Hysteroscopic septal resection with concurrent laparoscopy is the treatment of choice for symptomatic septate uterus. Unlike the transabdominal approach, it is a safe and effective method of achieving normal or near-normal uterus, in an outpatient setting. There is minimal risk of intrauterine adhesions with rapid recovery. With hysteroscopic metroplasty, patient can immediately plan conception postoperatively and has lower risk of uterine rupture during pregnancy when compared to abdominal approach, and vaginal delivery is possible, avoiding subsequent cesarean delivery.

References

1. Steinmetz GP. Formation of artificial vagina. West J Surg. 1940;48:169–3.
2. Zhu L, Wong F, Lang JH. Minimally invasive surgery and map for female genital abnormalities, vol. 150. Beijing: People's Medical Publishing House; 2010.
3. Cao ZY. Chinese J Obstet Gynecol. (clinical edition) Beijing: People's Medical Publishing House. 2010;374
4. Braun P, Grau FV, Pons RM, Enguix DP. Is hysterosalpingography able to diagnose all uterine malformations correctly? A retrospective study. Eur J Radiol. 2005;53:274–9.
5. Hannema SE, Hughes IA. Regulation of Wolffian duct development. Horm Res. 2007;67:142–51.

6. Acien P, Acien M, Sanchez-Ferrer M. Complex malformations of the female genital tract. New types and revision of classification. Hum Reprod. 2004;19:2377–84.
7. Oppelt P, von Have M, Paulsen M, Strissel P, Strick R, Brucker S, Wallwiener S, Beckmann M. Female genital malformations and their associated abnormalities. Fertil Steril. 2007;87:335–42.
8. The American Fertility Society classifications of adnexal adhesions, distal tubal occlusion, tubal occlusion secondary to tubal ligation, tubal pregnancies, müllerian anomalies and intrauterine adhesions. Fertil Steril. 1988;49(6):944–55.
9. Buttram VC Jr, Gibbons WE. Müllerian anomalies: a proposed classification. (An analysis of 144 cases). Fertil Steril. 1979;32(1):40–6.
10. Moutos MD, Damewood DM, Schlaff DW, Rock AJ. A comparison of the reproductive outcome between women with a unicornuate uterus and women with a didelphic uterus. Fertil Steril. 1983;58:88–93.
11. Buttram CV. Mullerian anomalies and their management. Fertil Steril. 1983;40:159–63.
12. Marcus S, Al-Shawaf T, Brinsden P. The obstetric outcome of in vitro fertilization and embryo transfer in women with congenital uterine malformation. Am J Obstet Gynecol. 1996;175:85–9.
13. Fedele L, Bianchi S. Hysteroscopic metroplasty for septate uterus. Obstet Gynecol Clin North Am. 1995;22:473–89.
14. Fedele L, Dorta M, Brioschi D, et al. Pregnancies in septate uteri: outcome in relation to site of uterine implantation as determined by sonography. Am J Roentgenol. 1989;152:781–4.
15. Dabirashrafi H, Bahadori M, Mohammad K, et al. Septate uterus: new idea on the histologic features of the septum in this abnormal uterus. Am J Obstet Gynecol. 1995;172:105–7.
16. Wu MH, Hsu CC, Huang KE. Detection of congenital müllerian duct anomalies using three-dimensional ultrasound. J Clin Ultrasound. 1997;25:487.
17. Jurkovic D, Geipel A, Gruboeck K, et al. Three-dimensional ultrasound for the assessment of uterine anatomy and detection of congenital anomalies: a comparison with hysterosalpingography and two-dimensional sonography. Ultrasound Obstet Gynecol. 1995;5:233.
18. Bermejo C, Martínez Ten P, Cantarero R, et al. Three-dimensional ultrasound in the diagnosis of Müllerian duct anomalies and concordance with magnetic resonance imaging. Ultrasound Obstet Gynecol. 2010;35:593.
19. Leung JW, Hricak H. Role of magnetic resonance imaging in the evaluation of gynecologic disease. In: Callen PW, editor. Ultrasonography in obstetrics and gynecology. 4th ed. Philadelphia, PA: WB Saunders; 2000. p. 940.
20. Soares SR, Barbosa dos Reis MM, Camargos AF. Diagnostic accuracy of sonohysterography, transvaginal sonography, and hysterosalpingography in patients with uterine cavity diseases. Fertil Steril. 2000;73:406.
21. Homer HA, Li TC, Cooke ID. The septate uterus: a review of management and reproductive outcome. Fertil Steril. 2000;73:1–14.
22. Taylor E, Gomel V. The uterus and fertility. Fertil Steril. 2008;89:1–16.
23. Pellerito JS, McCarthy SM, Doyle MB, et al. Diagnosis of uterine anomalies: relative accuracy of MR imaging, endovaginal sonography, and hysterosalpingography. Radiology. 1992;183:795.
24. Kupesic S. Clinical implications of sonographic detection of uterine anomalies for reproductive outcome. Ultrasound Obstet Gynecol. 2001;18:387–400.
25. March MC, Israel R. Hysteroscopic management of recurrent abortion caused by septate uterus. Am J Obstet Gynecol. 1987;156:834–42.
26. Rock A, Schlaff DW. The obstetric consequences of uterovaginal anomalies. Fertil Steril. 1985;43:681–91.
27. Heinonen PK, Saarikoski S, Pystynen P. Reproductive performance of women with uterine anomalies. An evaluation of 182 cases. Acta Obstet Gynecol Scand. 1982;61(2):157–62.
28. Simon C, Martinez L, Pardo F, et al. Mullerian defects in women with normal reproductive outcome. Fertil Steril. 1991;56(6):1192–3.
29. Fischetti SG, Politi G, Lomeo E, Garozzo G. Magnetic resonance in the evaluation of Mullerian duct anomalies. Radiol Med (Torino). 1995;89(1-2):105–11.

30. Daly CD, Maier D, Soto-Albors C. Hysteroscopic metroplasty: six years experience. Obstet Gynecol. 1989;73:201–5.
31. Römer T, Lober R. Hysteroscopic correction of a complete septate uterus using a balloon technique. Hum Reprod. 1997;12:478–9.
32. Donnez J, Nisolle M. Endoscopic laser treatment of uterine malformations. Hum Reprod. 1997;12(7):1381.
33. Fedele L, Bianchi S, Marchini M, Mezzopane R, Di Nola G, Tozzi L. Residual uterine septum of less than 1 cm after hysteroscopic metroplasty does not impair reproductive outcome. Hum Reprod. 1996;11(4):727–9.
34. Dabirashrafi H, Mohammad K, Moghadami-Tabrizi N, Zandinejad K, Moghadami-Tabrizi M. Is estrogen necessary after hysteroscopic incision of the uterine septum? J Am Assoc Gynecol Laparosc. 1996;3(4):623–5.
35. Barakat AJ. Association of unilateral renal agenesis and genital anomalies. Case Rep Clin Pract Rev. 2002;3:57–60.
36. Valle RF, Sciarra JJ. Hysteroscopic treatment of the septate uterus. Obstet Gynecol. 1986;67(2):253–7.
37. De Cherney AH, Russell JB, Graebe RA, Polan ML. Resectoscopic management of mullerian fusion defects. Fertil Steril. 1986;45(5):726–8.

Asherman's Syndrome and Hysteroscopy

Ruma Satwik

8.1 Introduction

Asherman's syndrome is an acquired clinical condition arising out of partial or complete uterine obliteration by intrauterine adhesions resulting in any one or more of the following: (a) menstrual irregularity characterized by hypomenorrhoea or amenorrhoea, (b) infertility, (c) pregnancy loss and (d) obstetric complications such as abnormal placental attachment and preterm labour. The name is acquired from the Israeli physician, John G. Asherman, who in 1948 clearly characterized this condition [1].

8.2 Prevalence of Asherman's Syndrome

The prevalence of Asherman's syndrome varies with patient demographics and the detection methods employed. In women with history of prior miscarriage, the incidence of intrauterine adhesions has been found to be between 6% and 31% [2, 3]. The incidence increases with the numbers of interventions for miscarriages being 16%, 14% and 31%, respectively, after one, two and three curettage procedures. The severity (filmy/dense) and extent of adhesions (judged by percentage of cavity obliteration) also increase with increasing number of interventions. The likelihood of adhesions forming is higher after a sharp curettage for missed abortion (31%) than for incomplete abortion (6%) [2]. In infertile women, undergoing hysteroscopy or HSG, the prevalence has been variously reported between 1.5% and 22% [4–10]. The variability may stem from clinician's awareness of the syndrome, criteria used for diagnosis, prevalence of genital infections or puerperal sepsis in a particular

R. Satwik, DGO, DNB, FNB (Reprod Med)
Centre of IVF and Human Reproduction, Institute of Obstetrics and Gynaecology,
Sir Gangaram Hospital, New Delhi, India

© Springer Nature Singapore Pte Ltd. 2018
S. Jain, D. B. Inamdar (eds.), *Manual of Fertility Enhancing Hysteroscopy*,
https://doi.org/10.1007/978-981-10-8028-9_8

geographic location and policy regarding use of sharp, blunt or suction curettages for evacuation of gravid uteri [11, 12].

The true incidence of Asherman's syndrome, however, may be unknown as milder degrees of obliteration may remain asymptomatic. Hence it is asserted that the term Asherman's syndrome be applied only to women having intrauterine adhesions that present with one or more of the aforementioned symptoms, namely: menstrual irregularity, infertility, pregnancy loss or placentation abnormalities. Asymptomatic intrauterine adhesions found incidentally should not be labelled as Asherman's syndrome [11, 12].

8.3   Aetiology

Incriminating factors have been surgeries on pregnant uterus, like vigorous uterine curettage especially for missed abortions (risk of uterine synechiae developing is 14–31%) [2, 3, 13, 14], post puerperal curettage (risk of synechiae developing, 25%) [15], diagnostic curettage (risk of synechiae developing, 1.6%), submucous myomectomy (risk of synechiae developing, 31–45%) [16], septal resection (risk of synechiae developing, 6.7%), caesarean sections (risk of synechiae developing, 2–2.8%) [17, 18], abdominal myomectomy with breach of cavity or misplaced sutures (1.3% of all cases of Asherman's) [17] or after endometrial infections like genital tuberculosis (17.5% in infertile women undergoing hysteroscopy) [19] and non-specific endometritis (35.4% of women undergoing hysteroscopic synechiolysis) [20] or after cavity radiation.

Auditing their own cases of 36 women that underwent an open myomectomy, Conforti et al. showed the presence of intrauterine adhesions in 50% of women undergoing open myomectomy 3 months after surgery when assessed by hysteroscopy. The risk of adhesions increased with increasing number of fibroids removed, but its incidence or severity was not influenced by an inadvertent uterine cavity breach [21].

8.4   Pathology

Asherman's syndrome occurs as the end result of healing by fibrosis of traumatized or inflamed endometrial surfaces. The basal layer of endometrium is responsible for regeneration of the functional layer. Trauma or inflammation to this layer results in poor regenerative capability and predisposes to endometrial healing by fibrosis, the hallmark lesion of this syndrome.

Fibrosis leads to the development of either *intrauterine adhesions* or *endometrial scarring*. Intrauterine adhesion is a fibrotic bridge between anterior and posterior uterine walls as a result of apposition of inflamed surfaces causing various degrees of cavity obliteration. Endometrial scarring, on the other hand, is a result of fibrosis within the walls presenting generally as thin hypovascularized endometrium, the cavity itself being more or less normal in volume. Since there could be subjectivity in interpreting the appearance of such endometria, scarring is best established by a combination of hysteroscopic appearance and a biopsy of the suspicious area showing the presence of fibrotic tissue [12]. In most cases, the two pathologies of intrauterine adhesions and endometrial scarring coexist.

Grossly, the adhesions could be *filmy* or *dense* or both. Filmy adhesions are ones that are easily broken by the hysteroscope. Dense adhesions cannot be broken by the hysteroscope and need a sharp mechanical or energy device for division. The adhesions could be *isolated* or *multiple* or *diffuse*, involving the entire cavity. They could be variously located and are classified either as *central* adhesions, *marginal* adhesions, *cornual* adhesions or *cervical* adhesions. The endometrial cavity could be completely or partially occluded by these adhesions. Adhesions only in the region of cervical os with the upper cavity being normal, present with cryptomenorrhoea and dysmenorrhoea.

Histologically, the sectioned endometrial tissue shows replacement of endometrial stroma by fibrous tissue and sometimes by calcified deposits. The distinction between the functional and basal layer of the endometrium is lost, and the entire thickness of endometrium is represented by an epithelial monolayer, which is non-responsive to hormonal stimulation. There is paucity of glands, which usually appear as inactive cubo-columnar epithelium of the endometrial type. Vessels of the thin-walled dilated type may predominate, but in most cases the tissue is avascular. The fibrosis may involve various depths of myometrium as well.

Other histopathological appearances may include necrotizing granulomatous lesions, caseating granulomas and foreign body granulomas based on its specific aetiology.

8.5   Classification

Most classification systems take into consideration the nature of adhesion as seen on hysteroscopy; and extent of cavity involvement as seen on hysteroscopy or hysterosalpingography (HSG), to stage the disease. March et al. [22] were one of the first groups to score intrauterine adhesions based on hysteroscopic appearance of the degree of uterine cavity involvement as minimal, less than one-fourth cavity obliterated; moderate, one-fourth to three-fourths cavity obliterated; and severe, greater than three-fourths cavity obliterated. Hamou et al. in 1983 [23] classified the disease based on the location of adhesions as isthmic, cornual, central or marginal. Valle and Sciarra in 1988 [24] described another classification system that took into account the degree of cavity obliteration and the histopathological type of adhesion i.e. whether made up of basal endometrial tissue, fibromuscular tissue or connective tissue. Although these systems objectively and precisely describe the severity of disease, they were criticized for being unable to prognosticate reproductive outcomes.

The American Fertility Society in 1988 developed an objective scoring system for staging Asherman's syndrome that correlated menstrual history with hysteroscopic and hysterosalpingographic findings [25] (Table 8.1). Based on this, the

Table 8.1 AFS Classification of intrauterine adhesions (1988) [25]

Feature	Extent		
Extent of cavity involved	<1/3	1/3–2/3	>2/3
Score	1	2	4
Type of adhesions	Filmy	Filmy and dense	Dense
Score	1	2	4
Menstrual pattern	Normal	Hypomenorrhoea	Amenorrhoea
Score	0	2	4

woman can be categorized as having stage 1 disease, if her score is between 1 and 4; stage 2, if her score is between 5 and 9; and stage 3, if her score is above 9. This classification, though good to prognosticate women with Asherman's, is still not universally used by practitioners across the world.

Prognostic Classification
Stage I: (mild) 1–4
Stage II: (moderate) 5–8
Stage III: (severe) >9

8.6   Clinical Symptoms

The most common symptom of Asherman's syndrome is menstrual dysfunction, which is seen in about 70% of women with intrauterine adhesions. Menstrual dysfunction manifests, in descending order of frequency, as hypomenorrhoea, secondary amenorrhoea and dysmenorrhoea. The most plausible reason here is loss of functional endometrium and its replacement with hormone-nonresponsive lining. Hormone replacement therapy does not correct this form of menstrual irregularity.

Infertility follows as a result of absence of sperm-egg interaction due to tubal ostial or cervical canal occlusion and as a result of poor interface available for implantation. Pregnancy occurs if implantation takes place on the anatomically preserved endometrial surface. However, increased rates of pregnancy loss have been seen from uteri affected by scarring as a result of poor overall vascularity [26].

Other pregnancy complications with Asherman's syndrome are tubal and cervical ectopics, defective placentation leading to intrauterine growth restriction, placenta accreta, antepartum and postpartum haemorrhage and preterm deliveries due to space restriction (Table 8.2).

8.7   Diagnosis of Intrauterine Adhesions

The methods for diagnosis of intrauterine adhesions may be regarded as belonging to one of the two categories: methods requiring cervical canulation, such as hysterosalpingography (HSG), sonosalpingography (SSG) and hysteroscopy, and methods not requiring cervical canulation like transvaginal sonography (TVS) or magnetic resonance imaging (MRI). In general, the cervical canulation methods are invasive

Table 8.2 Frequency of clinical symptoms seen in Asherman's syndrome [14]

Clinical symptom	Frequency (%)
Hypomenorrhoea	31
Amenorrhoea	37
Dysmenorrhoea	3.5
Infertility	43
Pregnancy Loss	40
Placenta accreta	13
Preterm deliveries	23
Ectopic pregnancy	12

in nature but deemed superior to the ones not requiring canulation in terms of their diagnostic ability. However, in cases of cervical canal obliteration, the other methods may be adopted.

8.7.1 HSG

Hysterosalpingography is a simple screening method for intrauterine adhesions in infertile patients. Intrauterine adhesions appear as sharply defined filling defects, sometimes with significant cavity obliteration (Figs. 8.1 and 8.2). In addition, it provides crucial information about fallopian tubal patency, course and contour. However, HSG has a number of limitations. Firstly, it has a poor sensitivity for detection of minor adhesions since filmy adhesions might not consistently produce abnormal shadows on HSG. Also, an excessive amount of contrast medium in the uterus can obliterate shadows caused by even sturdier intrauterine adhesions. And, it may not detect endometrial fibrosis per se. Secondly, HSG has a high false-positive rate (PPV of 50%) [27], since air bubbles, mucous and debris may all mimic filling defects. Also, poor placement of the cannula can cause intravasation that may be interpreted to be due to endometritis. Thirdly, it does not define the nature of intrauterine adhesion and hence cannot be used to score the lesion prognostically.

8.7.2 Ultrasound

In women with severe intrauterine adhesions, ultrasonography may show the following typical appearance: the endometrial echo becomes difficult to visualize, with irregular thickness and one or more interruptions of the endometrium at the sites of fibrosis. In addition, there may sometimes be one or more echo-lucent areas interrupting the endometrium, representing localized collection of menstrual blood in an area where the functional layers of the endometrium are preserved.

Both the sensitivity and the specificity of ultrasound in diagnosis of intrauterine adhesions have been reported to be quite low (52% and 11%, respectively) [28, 29]. Nevertheless, ultrasonography is useful when HSG is not possible because of obliteration of lower uterine cavity. In this situation, ultrasonography may be used to evaluate the upper uterine cavity, and the findings may be of prognostic significance. A mid-cycle transvaginal sonography is often ordered after a corrective

Fig. 8.1 Right marginal and fundal synechiae on HSG with bilateral tubal block (Courtesy: Dr. K K Saxena, Department of Radiology, Sir Ganga Ram Hospital, New Delhi)

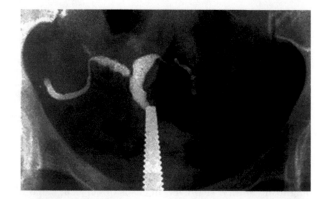

Fig. 8.2 Central synechiae with bilateral spill on HSG (Courtesy: Dr K K Saxena, Department of Radiology, Sir Ganga Ram Hospital, New Delhi)

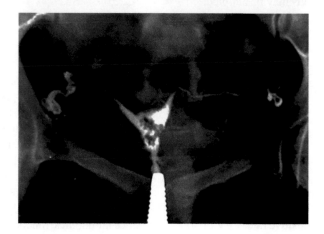

procedure for Asherman's syndrome to assess the functionality of endometrium in terms of thickness, pattern and vascularity, a unique ability, which the other modalities are unable to do.

Three-dimensional ultrasonography techniques have been used by a few investigators to detect adhesions in the uterine cavity, with a better sensitivity (85%) and specificity (45%) when comparing against 3D sonohysterography [28].

8.7.3   Sonohysterography

It involves transvaginal sonography (TVS) after intrauterine injection of isotonic saline using paediatric Foley's catheter number 8 and checking on TVS to see if any lesions are visible in the distended uterine cavity. It is considered a simple, cheap, effective, easily available and minimally invasive method for detection of intrauterine adhesions. Adhesions are suspected if one or more echogenic areas are seen between the anterior and posterior walls in the liquid-filled uterine cavity. Diagnostic accuracy for detection of intrauterine adhesions is similar to that of HSG. In a review of all studies done on the subject from 1950 till July 2014, an excellent pooled sensitivity of 82% and a specificity of 99% have been reported when compared against the gold standard of hysteroscopy [30].

8.7.4 Hysteroscopy

Is the gold standard procedure for diagnosis of intrauterine adhesions against which other investigative modalities are measured. It not only diagnoses but also defines their nature and extent as well while offering the choice of concurrent treatment. Filmy adhesions appear the same as the surrounding endometrium, whereas myomatous or fibrous adhesions may appear thick and white. Adhesions may be vascular or avascular depending upon whether they are myomatous or fibrous. Endometrial fibrosis appears as pale patches. The adhesions need to be classified based on their exact location. They can either be *central*, ones in the cavity and with free space intervening between the adhesion and the lateral wall, or *marginal*, ones with no intervening space, cornual or cervico-isthmic [31].

Hysteroscopy has one disadvantage over non-invasive procedures, in that, with complete canal occlusion or with severe cavity obliteration, upper cavity assessment may become difficult, especially in unskilled hands.

8.7.5 MRI

May be ordered when negotiating the cervix becomes impossible either during HSG, SSG or hysteroscopy [32]. It allows the visualization of upper cavity and the assessment of residual functional endometrium. Based on this assessment a hysteroscopic corrective procedure may be undertaken or abandoned. The adhesions on MRI appear hypo-intense when compared to surrounding tissues (Table 8.3) [33].

8.8 Treatment of Asherman's Syndrome

Asherman's syndrome can be a very difficult condition to treat. Many treatment modalities like expectant management, medical management and surgical management have been tried with surgery forming the mainstay of treatment.

8.8.1 Expectant Management

Expectant management basically involves following up cases over a period of time to see if some or all symptoms are relieved. Schenker and Margalioth in 1982 [17] describe a series of 23 women with amenorrhea, 18 of whom in the absence of any intervention resumed spontaneous menses in a span of 1–7 years after

Table 8.3 Comparison of various methods used for diagnosing intrauterine adhesions

	Sensitivity	Specificity/PPV	Advantages	Limitations	References
Hysteroscopy	100	100	Allows characterization of lesion and concurrent correction	Skill based, invasive, expensive	
HSG	75–79%	50–60%	Simple, safe, minimally invasive, cheap. Assesses tubal patency too	Misses minor adhesions, overdiagnoses in presence of air, polyp	Soares et al. [27] Raziel et al. [103]
TVS	52%	0–11%	Assesses functional endometrium, myometrial, adnexal pathology	Poor sensitivity and specificity	Soares et al. [27] Salle et al. [29] Sylvestre et al. [28]
SSG	75–82%	42.5–99%	Assesses functional endometrium, myometrial, adnexal pathology	Equal sensitivity, specificity to HSG	Soares et al. [27] Seshadri et al. [30]
3D sonography	87% Compared to 3D-SSG	45% Compared to 3D-SSG	Assesses functional endometrium, myometrial, adnexal pathology	Not always available, expensive	Sylvestre et al. [28]
MRI	NA	NA	Allows assessment of residual endometrium when hysteroscopy is not possible	expensive	Letterie et al. [32]

detection. In the same review, they come across a set of 292 women, identified with Asherman's syndrome and infertility, 133 (45.5%) of whom conceived spontaneously in the same follow-up period of 1–7 years. It is not clear through this review whether the women who conceived or resumed their menstrual function had lesser or severe degree of the disease. But what can be said with certainty is that some women with Asherman's syndrome, perhaps the ones afflicted to a lesser degree, are likely to conceive spontaneously over a period of time.

8.8.2   Traditional Methods

Traditionally, the treatment advocated for Asherman's syndrome was cervical dilatation [1] (that breaks cervical canal adhesions) and/or uterine curettage (that breaks cavity adhesions) [34] followed by insertion of intrauterine device/Foley's catheter and oral oestrogen therapy [35, 36]. Other traditional therapies have involved manual breaking of intrauterine adhesions after hysterotomy or the very radical treatment: hysterectomy, if the patient had cryptomenorrhoea and dysmenorrhoea [35]. However, all these treatments were either blind or too invasive, lead to a higher degree of complications like uterine perforations and did not give consistent results in women desiring fertility.

8.8.3   Hysteroscopic Lysis of Intrauterine Adhesions (Synechiolysis) (Fig. 8.3a–f)

The modern-day treatment of Asherman's syndrome, hence, relies exclusively on hysteroscopic methods, which involve lysis of adhesions under direct vision without having to open the abdomen. The principles of treatment remain (1) restoring full uterine capacity, (2) undertaking measures to prevent recurrence that include prevention of apposition of freshly dissected surface and early re-epithelialization and (3) the development of functional endometrium.

Amongst the early users of hysteroscopy for treatment of Asherman's syndrome were Levine and Neuwirth [37] who in 1973 described simultaneous use of laparoscopy and hysteroscopy to lyse intrauterine adhesions. Subsequent comparative and descriptive studies proved hysteroscopic lysis to be superior over traditional methods [22, 38–41]. Hysteroscopic lysis of adhesions has since seen major improvements in all aspects including the optics, dimension and flexibility of endoscopes, instruments and energy sources used and methods used for guidance in completely obliterated cavities.

8.8.3.1 Principles of hysteroscopic Synechiolysis

Some principles during hysteroscopic lysis are to be made note of

1. It helps to inform the patient with severe adhesions that one procedure may not suffice in restoring uterine capacity and that one or more repeat procedures may be needed [42]. Indeed, the immediate goal of restoration of uterine capacity is met when both ostia are visualized in the same plane and more than one procedure

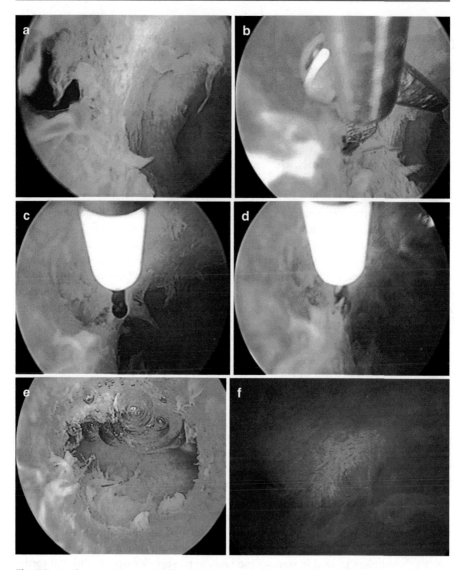

Fig. 8.3 (**a**) Central adhesion. (**b**) Synechiolysis using scissors. (**c**) Marginal adhesion being lysed with bipolar twizzle. (**d**) Marginal adhesion being lysed with bipolar twizzle. (**e**) Cavity after lysis of right lateral synechia. The point of synechial detachment can be seen on the anterior wall. (**f**) Right fundo-cornual adhesion

may be needed to safely achieve that. More than ten repeat procedures have been described in women with severe Asherman's syndrome to restore uterine volume and shape [43].

2. Although *office* hysteroscopy for operative procedures has been attempted with reasonable patient satisfaction and procedure completion rates [44], this author believes there is limited role of office hysteroscopy in synechiolysis. It is best

done in the operating room under general anaesthesia in order to maximize operator ease and minimize patient discomfort and complications.

3. If a concomitant tubal patency test is planned, perform it prior to beginning synechiolysis, since methylene blue test after lysis could be falsely negative, due to intravasation caused by dye entering into opened sinuses. Also the pressure of dye may rupture the uterus at weakened areas created during lysis. Ensure that the dye is light in colour so that it does not stain the endometrium deeply and make subsequent visualization difficult.

4. In case of complete cavity obliteration, the above may be irrelevant.

5. Lysis begins and proceeds in a caudo-cephalad direction. Start with the thinner and central adhesions first, so as to enhance working space and visualization. Thick central adhesions are lysed next. Marginal and cornual adhesions are more difficult to treat [31] and should be dealt with in the end.

6. Thin adhesions may break with fluid distension or with blunt force applied with the hysteroscope itself. Moderate to severe adhesions require special instruments.

7. While lysing marginal adhesions, injury to major vessels is possible and this may be difficult to control. A laparoscopic control is helpful in defining the limits of dissection, thus preventing perforation and vessel injury.

8. The adhesion reformation frequency is dependent upon the site of original adhesions. Central adhesions have the least rate of recurrence. Cornual adhesions, marginal adhesions and cervico-isthmic adhesions are prone to recurring with a higher frequency [31].

8.8.3.2 Instruments for Synechiolysis

There are two kinds of instruments in use: ones using mechanical energy like scissors and the others using energy sources such as diathermy or laser. Mechanical instruments include the 4–5 Fr semirigid scissors which cut via sharp dissection or the biopsy forceps which lyses by blunt force. Energy instruments are precise and effective and use either monopolar or bipolar current or laser for vaporization and lysis. Monopolar instruments include resectoscopic Collin's knife (Fig. 8.4b) or the Bugbee monopolar electrode (Fig. 8.5) [45, 46]. Bipolar energy-using device is the Versapoint electrosurgical system, which has proven its efficacy and safety in synechiolysis [47]. Bipolar systems use saline as a distending medium thus minimizing complications associated with water intoxication. Nd:YAG laser [48], KTP laser [49] and diode laser [50] have all been utilized for vaporization and lysis of intrauterine adhesions with reasonable results. In general, mechanical devices like scissors and forceps are considered safer than the energy devices. Firstly, the energy devices, due to their collateral spread, can theoretically damage the normal endometrium, and secondly, greater risk of injury to viscera exists with them in cases of perforation. However, the ease of lysis is greater with energy devices. They are quite efficient in dividing marginal adhesions, which are difficult to reach with rigid scissors. Other advantage is the simultaneous haemostasis possible with energy instruments and hence the availability of a clearer field during surgery.

Fig. 8.4 (**a**) Monopolar
electrodes: cutting loop
and ball electrode. (**b**)
Monopolar electrodes:
Collin's knife

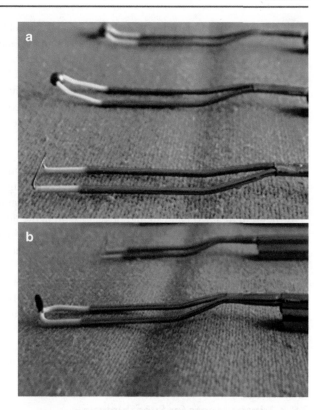

Fig. 8.5 Bugbee
monopolar electrode

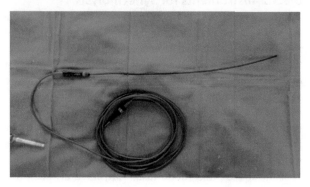

It is important to be wary of complications that may arise due to the use of electrical energy or laser. These can be minimized by using the lowest current setting possible, needle electrode instead of a loop electrode, and avoiding vigorous application of energy at the fundus or the cornua.

8.8.3.3 Approach in Severe Adhesions
Since hysteroscopy cannot view the depth of adhesion, dissection is often limited by a fear of perforation or major organ injury. This becomes an impediment especially

in cases with complete or near-complete cavity obliteration. Additional guidance methods help and several such have been defined.

Laparoscopic guidance: This technique appears to be effective and safe for the reconstruction of a functional endometrial cavity in women with complete or near-complete obliteration of uterine cavity [51–53]. Laparoscopy is expected to warn surgeons of an impending perforation when extreme thinning of myometrium as evidenced by wall translucency or herniation is observed. But this approach could literally be cutting it too thin, and perforations are known to occur even with laparoscopic guidance. Its best use is then in early recognition and treatment of such perforations.

Ultrasound guidance: By defining the limits of fundus and the lateral uterine walls, real-time transabdominal ultrasound guidance reduces complications such as perforations while allowing for a more complete procedure, thus reducing reoperation rates [54–56]. Ultrasound guidance has been deemed to be less expensive, less invasive and more effective in reducing intraoperative perforations than laparoscopic guidance [53]. A combined approach using simultaneous transabdominal and transrectal ultrasound probes has also been described for guidance during hysteroscopic synechiolysis in patients with simultaneous obliteration of the cervical canal [57].

Fluoroscopically guided approach: Fluoroscopic guidance enables a radiologic view of pockets of endometrium behind an otherwise blind-ending hysteroscopic view. A spinal needle through which radiographic contrast material is injected is used in parallel to the hysteroscope to help outline pockets of normal endometrium beyond an obliterating adhesion and thus guide synechiolysis. Images of the hysteroscope are coordinated with those on an image intensifier. Thomson et al. in 2007 report on a series of 30 patients so treated, 96% of whom, with AFS grade 1–3 Asherman's, regained menstruation and 56% got pregnant. Mean operative time was reported to be 46 min [58]. An obvious limitation of this method seems to be the need of an image intensifier and a radiographer in the operation theatre, which is not always possible in low-resource settings. Another limitation might be the unnecessary exposure to radiation.

Other methods: Other methods described in literature that guide dissection include but are not limited to (1) the use of laparoscopic transfundal injection of methylene blue dye [59], which selectively stains the endometrium leaving the myometrium and fibrotic tissue unstained; (2) myometrial scoring method [24], where a Collin's knife is used to make six to eight 4 mm deep, vertical incisions, on the walls of the narrowed uterus to enable widening of the cavity on which a functional endometrium is expected to grow; (3) blind use of cervical dilator in a completely obliterated uterus to create two lateral passages and a central fibrous septum which is then excised hysteroscopically [53]; and (4) use of IUCD placed during primary surgery for guidance during second-look surgery [60]. Although the investigators, in all these series, have reported success in terms of cavity restoration, menses resumption and pregnancies, these procedures have not been clinically validated in other centres and hence cannot be recommended in standard practice.

8.9   Complications

Adverse events linked to hysteroscopic synechiolysis can be immediate or late. The most common immediate events are intravasation of distension fluid and its attending complications, uterine perforation and haemorrhage. Late events are adhesion reformation and risk of uterine rupture during a subsequent pregnancy. The complication rate depends on the complexity of the procedure, the time taken for surgery and the operator's experience.

8.9.1   Haemorrhage

The risk of significant haemorrhage is higher with adhesiolysis than with other operative hysteroscopic procedures (relative risk 5.5), although the average absolute risk for synechiolysis has been described to vary from 0.6% to 6% [61, 62]. Whenever identified, it can be controlled with needle/ball electrode (Fig. 8.6) cauterization, Foley's bulb insertion (inflated with 10–20 mL of saline) for 24 h and, in some cases, uterine artery ligation through the vaginal route. In two cases with significant haemorrhage on days 4 and 18 postoperatively, high doses of intravenous oestrogen use (25 mg CEE in 50 mL normal saline over 20 min every 6 h) have been described to successfully control bleeding by promoting epithelialization [63].

8.9.2   Perforation

Hysteroscopic synechiolysis also stands the highest risk for perforation when compared to other hysteroscopic procedures (relative risk between 7 and 9). The absolute risk of perforation stands at 1.6–4.5% [64, 65]. Most perforations are entry

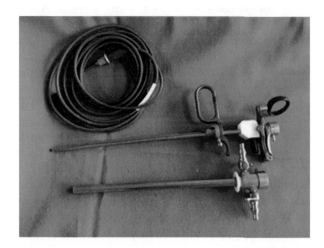

Fig. 8.6 Resectoscope through which the Collin's knife, monopolar needle or ball electrodes are inserted for various purposes such as synechiolysis, haemostasis etc

related, and others occur during synechiolysis, more with use of electrocautery than with scissors. Once recognized, a laparoscopy should be performed to look for haemorrhage and visceral injuries. If found, abnormal haemorrhage should be controlled either with pressure, cauterization or application of haemostatic sutures. Visceral injuries may need a laparotomy.

8.9.3 Fluid Overload

Most reports of complications arising out of fluid intravasation and overload have occurred with hysteroscopic myomectomy procedures although it can occur with a lesser frequency but equal severity in women undergoing synechiolysis as well [66]. Same is dealt with elsewhere in the book.

8.9.4 Risk of Recurrence

One of the main challenges of treating Asherman's syndrome is the risk of adhesion reformation. Recurrence rates are known to range from 0% to 15% with mild adhesions, 16–38% with moderate adhesions and 42–80% with severe adhesions [67, 68]. Location of intrauterine adhesions too has a significant bearing on adhesion reformation with recurrence rates of 68% with central, 87% with marginal, 82% with cornual and 100% with cervico-isthmic synechiae described in a well-designed prospective study [68].

8.9.5 Uterine Rupture During a Subsequent Pregnancy

This risk has been ascertained to be the highest with hysteroscopic metroplasties. Uterine perforation and use of electro-excision add to the risk [44].

8.10 Prevention of Adhesion Reformation

With such high rates of recurrence quoted above, one cannot underscore enough the need for effective measures to reduce that risk. Anti-adhesion therapy so far used aims to either create a physical barrier between the raw unhealed apposing uterine surfaces or promote early re-epithelialization of denuded surfaces. To achieve the former, the measures described in medical literature are *intrauterine device*, *Foley's catheter bulb* and *biodegradable adhesion barriers*. To achieve the latter effect, *high-dose oestrogen therapy* mostly and *amnion grafts* occasionally have been employed. One other method using serial mechanical breakage of synechiae has been described too.

8.10.1 Serial Mechanical Breakage of Synechiae

Robinson et al. [69] performed serial office-based hysteroscopies starting 2 weeks after the primary procedure, in women with moderate to severe Asherman's syndrome, to lyse any reformed adhesions bluntly using the hysteroscope. Subsequent procedures were undertaken 1–3 weeks after the second procedure, till no disease was seen. All procedures were performed in the outpatient department in the absence of general or local anaesthesia and without cervical dilatation. A mean of three visits, with a maximum of ten, were required to achieve an overall improvement in their mean adhesion scores, and 92% of women (22/24) were able to do so. Thirty percent of women attained full-term pregnancies and deliveries. One drawback of this procedure might be the disinclination of women to undergo as many procedures. Also this study was uncontrolled, hence inconclusive regarding its true efficacy against a control population.

8.10.2 Intrauterine Device

Placement of intrauterine device (IUD) after synechiolysis has been the standard therapy to prevent adhesion recurrence [36, 70–72]. Literature abounds in the use of various types of IUDs post synechiolysis including the Lippes loop [44, 69, 73, 74], the Duck foot and the butterfly device [75] and the copper T and progesterone-releasing devices. While Lippes loop is favoured by most authors due to its inert nature and its rather large surface area, copper-bearing and progesterone-releasing IUDs have fallen out of favour due to their small surface area and copper's ability to induce excessive inflammation [76, 77]. Others are not in consistent use due to lack of universal availability. Small RCTs conducted in the past 25 years have shown mixed results with respect to adhesion reformation [78, 79]. A small prospective interventional study [80] on the effectiveness of IUDs in adhesion prevention after septoplasty found that adhesions developed in 5.3%, 12%, 10.5% and 0% of the untreated, IUD + oestrogen-treated, IUD-only-treated and oestrogen-only-treated women, respectively. None of the differences, however, were significant. Regarding pregnancy, the differences between groups were also not significant. The adhesion reformation rates with IUD have been reported up to 35% [81]. As of now strong evidence to recommend an IUD after synechiolysis does not exist.

8.10.3 Intrauterine Balloon

The use of a balloon to prevent adhesion formation after adhesiolysis helps by creating a physical barrier between opposing uterine walls to prevent their adhesion. Investigators have used paediatric Foley's catheter numbers 8–10 inflated with 3–10 mL of saline, for up to 5–14 days. The biggest criticisms of its use are increased risk of ascending infection from the vagina, decreased blood flow to uterine walls from pressure of the overinflated balloon with potential effects on endometrial regeneration and significant patient discomfort. A single report of spontaneous uterine rupture following intrauterine balloon post synechiolysis exists too [82]. As with the IUD, mixed results of balloon placement in adhesion prevention have been reported in both controlled and uncontrolled studies [79, 83–87].

8.10.4 Amnion Grafts

In patients with moderate to severe adhesions, fresh amnion grafts have been applied to the uterine cavity post synechiolysis with the aid of inflated Foley's catheter balloon for 2 weeks [88]. Adhesion reformation rates of 48% have been reported at 4 months, all of them being mild adhesions. Pregnancy rates of 26.7% vs. 13.3% were achieved, with and without the use of amnion graft in a small RCT [89]. Miscarriage rates of 60% were seen in the group achieving pregnancy, bringing the live birth down to 10% with use of amnion graft. The difference in pregnancy rates, miscarriage rates and live birth rates were not significant in groups using and not using amnion grafts.

8.10.5 Biodegradable Adhesion Barriers

Auto cross-linked hyaluronic acid [90], or hyaluronic acid in combination with carboxymethylcellulose and/or alginate [91], has been used in the form of gels [91, 92] or films [92] for prevention of postsurgical synechiae. Hyaluronic acid with carboxymethylcellulose is a well-known anti-adhesive material with long-lasting action for about 7 days that is used to separate abutting tissue surfaces. In a systematic review that pools the results of five studies reporting on the use of barrier gels, Bosteels et al. [93] concluded that any one of the barrier gels may be used following operative hysteroscopy in infertile women for decreasing recurrence of adhesions. The use of any barrier gel is associated with less severe de novo adhesions (RR 0.65, 95% CI 0.45–0.93, $p = 0.02$, 5 studies, 372 women, very low-quality evidence). The number needed to treat to benefit is 9. The mean reduction in adhesion scores is also significant (mean difference, -1.44, 95% CI -1.83 to -1.05, $p < 0.00001$, 1 study, 24 women); this benefit is even larger in women undergoing operative hysteroscopy for intrauterine adhesions (MD -3.30, 95% CI -3.43 to -3.17, $p < 0.00001$, 1 study, 19 women). Nevertheless, at present, no evidence for higher live birth or pregnancy rates exists with their use (risk ratio, 3.0, 95% confidence interval 0.35–26, $p = 0.32$, 1 study, 30 women, very low-quality evidence).

8.10.6 Oestrogen Progesterone Treatment

Oestrogen therapy in the treatment of Asherman's syndrome has been around for about six decades [94]. It works on the assumption that endometrial stromal and epithelial cells are oestrogen responsive, and exogenous oestrogen replacement in large doses after hysteroscopic synechiolysis would cause early endometrial epithe-lialization preventing adhesions between apposing surfaces [95]. Although its role in enhancing endometrial thickness and volume has been demonstrated following its use in women undergoing surgical abortion [96], literature does not concur on its benefit in preventing adhesions.

Estradiol valerate, 4 mg/day in divided doses for 21 days, with the addition of 10 mg medroxyprogesterone acetate once daily from day 15 to day 21 of oestrogen, has been the most common regimen used for this purpose. However, wide variations exist with respect to drug, dose, route of administration and the length of treatment. Estradiol valerate up to 12 mg/day has been given for 21–60 days. Conjugated equine oestrogens have been used in doses of 0.625–5 mg/day alone or in combina-tion with progesterone for up to 21–60 days. Dawood et al. [97] have used vaginal oestrogen 8 mg/day in divided doses for 28 days with oral micronized progesterone 100 mg/day added in the last 7 days for prevention of intrauterine adhesions. Despite years of use, few RCTs exist on its efficacy comparing it to placebo or other mea-sures, in preventing adhesions. In two comparative studies separated in time and space, Roy et al. [98] and Vercellini et al. [79] found no difference in adhesion ref-ormation rates on second-look hysteroscopy in women undergoing septal resection with oestrogen replacement therapy versus without. Yu et al. [85] found that the use of postoperative oestrogen therapy, IUD or intrauterine balloon did not appear to have any benefit in reducing the incidence of postoperative intrauterine adhesion formation over no treatment. Tonguc et al. in a similar tri-armed comparative study found no difference in effect between oestrogen use, IUD use and a placebo [81].

8.10.7 Results with Anti-adhesion Therapy

Despite years of studies evaluating prevention strategies for intrauterine adhesion formation after operative hysteroscopy, it is still unclear which strategies are most effective. That may be because good-quality data from multiple, unbiased, large, randomized controlled studies that report on parameters such as live births is still lacking that can recommend for or against their use. Two large recent reviews [99, 100] on the subject of anti-adhesion therapy following hysteroscopic synechiolysis found no evidence of a difference in live birth rates but did find low-quality evi-dence to suggest a significantly lower rate of adhesion reformation vis-à-vis placebo or no treatment (OR 0.36, 95% CI 0.20–0.64, p value = 0.0005, 7 studies, 528 women).

8.11 Outcomes of Treatment in Women with Asherman's Syndrome

Treatment outcomes in Asherman's syndrome should be determined based on the treatment indication. An immediate outcome of course remains cavity restoration, but that alone does not ensure treatment success, which is equally dependent upon attainment of functional endometrium especially in cases presenting with subfertility. In hormonally replete women, endometrial fibrosis is the chief cause of a nonfunctioning endometrium. Endometrial fibrosis is not amenable to surgery. Hence the degree of cavity restoration cannot be a measure of treatment success. Treatment outcomes in this section are described based on reproductive outcomes.

8.11.1 Reproductive Outcomes of Surgery for Asherman's Syndrome

While conception in women with untreated Asherman's syndrome is not unknown, a meticulous hysteroscopic lysis is known to improve these rates.

Before the use of hysteroscopy, the pregnancy rate after conventional treatment was reported to be 51% (540 out of 1052), which was only slightly better than found in those who had not been treated (133 out of 292; 46%) [17]. Hysteroscopic lysis improved these rates not only in infertile women, from 28.7% before surgery to 53.6% after hysteroscopic treatment [101], but also in women with two or more previous pregnancy losses; the live birth rate improved from 18.3% preoperatively to 68.6% postoperatively [102]. Subsequently, various studies done over the past 10 years have published their data on various reproductive outcomes like clinical pregnancy rates ranging from 40% to 60%, miscarriage rates from 11% to 22%, live birth rates ranging from 20% to 55%, term delivery rates of 75–95% of those conceived and antepartum haemorrhage due to placental attachment abnormality in the range of 2–25% of all live births (Table 8.4).

Overall, it can be said that hysteroscopic synechiolysis results in acceptable rates of pregnancy and live births in women suffering from Asherman's syndrome and infertility. These pregnancies however need to be carefully monitored, as the incidence of preterm births and placental attachment abnormalities is higher than in the general population.

Conclusions

Asherman's syndrome is a significant cause for infertility as well as menstrual disturbances and pregnancy complications. It results from endometrial trauma resulting from uterine surgeries or from endometritis that damages the basal endometrial layer irreversibly. Hysteroscopic synechiolysis is the primary method of treatment. Blunt, sharp and energy source linked lyses have all been used to obtain the goal of achieving full uterine capacity. One has to be wary of both immediate and late complications associated with lysis in severe cases. Ancillary methods adopted for prevention of adhesion reformation might be successful in reducing the risk and severity of adhesion reformation, but evidence is lacking on their efficacy in improving reproductive outcomes. Reproductive outcomes are mostly improved after hysteroscopic synechiolysis. Future research should focus on more effective ways to prevent adhesion reformation and on therapies to help regenerate functional endometrium.

Table 8.4 Reproductive outcomes after hysteroscopic synechiolysis

Study	Subjects 'N'	Treatment method	Pregnancy achieved (% of those attempting pregnancy)	Miscarriage rates (% of those conceived)	Live births (% of those attempting pregnancy)	Preterm births (% of live births)	Antepartum haemorrhage
Thomson AJ et al. 2007 [59]	30 (both infertility and RPL)	Fluoroscopic-guided hysteroscopic lysis	53% (9/17)	13.2%	46% (8/17)	25% (2/8)	25% (2/8)
Yu D et al. 2008 [68]	72 with infertility		43% overall (31/72) (62% mild, 45% moderate, 33% severe)	22.6%	33.3% overall (24/72) (43.75% mild, 30% moderate 16.7% severe)	5/19 (26.3%)	5/19 (26.3%)
Roy KK 2010 [99]	89 (not specified)	Hysteroscopic monopolar electrode knife	40.4% overall (58% mild, 30% moderate, 33% severe)	14%	34.74%	NA	12.5%
March CM 2011 [104]	1240	Hysteroscopic scissors	61.6% (764/1240)	11.8%	54.35% (674/1240)	7% (47/674)	1.9% (13/674)
Bhandari S et al. 2015 [105]	60 (not specified)	Hysteroscopic scissors	26.67% (16/60) overall (53% mild, 27% mod. 9.5% severe)	18.75%	21.67% (13/60)	3/13 (23.07%)	1/13 (7.7%)
Chen L 2017 [106]	357 with infertility	Hysteroscopic scissors. Bipolar Versapoint occasionally	48.2% overall (61% mild 53% moderate 25% severe)	15.15%	40.9% (140/352)	3.6% (5/140)	4.3% (6/140)

References

1. Asherman JG. Amenorrhoea traumatica. BJOG. 1948;55(11):23–30.
2. Adoni A, Palti Z, Milwidsky A, Dolberg M. The incidence of intrauterine adhesions following spontaneous abortion. Int J Fertil. 1982;27(2):117–8.
3. Friedler S, Margalioth EJ, Kafka I, Yaffe H. Incidence of post-abortion intra-uterine adhesions evaluated by hysteroscopy—a prospective stud. Hum Reprod. 1993;8(3):442–4.
4. Stillman RJ, Asarkof N. Association between Mullerian duct malformations and Asherman syndrome in infertile women. Obstet Gynecol. 1985;65:673–7.
5. La Sala GB, Montanari R, Dessanti L, Cigarini C, Sartori F. The role of diagnostic hysteroscopy and endometrial biopsy in assisted reproductive technologies. Fertil Steril. 1998;70:378–80.
6. Nawroth F, Foth D, Schmidt T. Minihysteroscopy as routine diagnostic procedure in women with primary infertility. J Am Assoc Gynecol Laparosc. 2003;10:396–8.
7. Hinckley MD, Milki AA. 1000 office-based hysteroscopies prior to in vitro fertilization: feasibility and findings. JSLS. 2004;8:103–7.
8. Yucebilgin MS, Aktan E, Bozkurt K, Kazandi M, Akercan F, Mgoyi L, Terek MC. Comparison of hydrosonography and diagnostic hysteroscopy in the evaluation of infertile patients. Clin Exp Obstet Gynecol. 2004;31:56–8.
9. Taylor PJ, Cumming DC, Hill PJ. Significance of intrauterine adhesions detected hysteroscopically in eumenorrheic infertile women and role of antecedent curettage in their formation. Am J Obstet Gynecol. 1981;139:239–42.
10. Preutthipan S, Linasmita V. A prospective comparative study between hysterosalpingography and hysteroscopy in the detection of intrauterine pathology in patients with infertility. J Obstet Gynaecol Res. 2003;29:33–7.
11. Deans R, Abbott J. Review of intrauterine adhesions. J Minim Invasive Gynecol. 2010;17(5):555–69.
12. Yu D, Wong Y, Cheong Y, Xia E, Li T. Asherman's syndrome. One century later. Fertil Steril. 2008;89(4):759–79.
13. Hooker AB, Lemmers M, Thurkow AL, Heymans MW, Opmeer BC, Brölmann HA, Mol BW, Huirne JA. Systematic review and meta-analysis of intrauterine adhesions after miscarriage: prevalence, risk factors and long-term reproductive outcome. Hum Reprod Update. 2014;20(2):262–78.
14. Hooker A, Fraenk D, Brölmann H, Huirne J. Prevalence of intrauterine adhesions after termination of pregnancy: a systematic review. Eur J Contracept Reprod Health Care. August 1, 2016;21(4):329–35.
15. Buttram UC, Turati G. Uterine synechiae: variation in severity and some conditions which may be conductive to severe adhesions. Int J Fertil. 1977;22:98–103.
16. Taskin O, Sadik S, Onoglu A, Gokdeniz R, Erturan E, Burak F, Wheeler JM. Role of endometrial suppression on the frequency of intrauterine adhesions after resectoscopic surgery. J Am Assoc Gynecol Laparosc. 2000;7:351–4.
17. Schenker JG, Margalioth EJ. Intrauterine adhesions: an updated appraisal. Fertil Steril. 1982;37:593–610.
18. Roge P, d'Ercole C, Cravello L, Boubli L, Blanc B. Hysteroscopic treatment of uterine synechias. A report of 102 cases. J Gynecol Obstet Biol Reprod (Paris). 1996;25:33–40.
19. Gupta N, Sharma JB, Mittal S, Singh N, Misra R, Kukreja M. Genital tuberculosis in Indian infertility patients. Int J Gynaecol Obstet. 2007;97(2):135–8.
20. Chen Y, Liu L, Luo Y, Chen M, Huan Y, Fang R. Prevalence and impact of chronic endometritis in patients with intrauterine adhesions: a prospective cohort study. J Minim Invasive Gynecol. 2017;24(1):74–9.
21. Conforti A, Krishnamurthy GB, Dragamestianos C, Kouvelas S, Micallef Fava A, Tsimpanakos I, Magos A. Intrauterine adhesions after open myomectomy: an audit. Eur J Obstet Gynecol Reprod Biol. 2014;179:42–5.

22. March CM, Israel R. Intrauterine adhesions secondary to elective abortion. Hysteroscopic diagnosis and management. Obstet Gynecol. 1976;48(4):422–4.
23. Hamou J, Salat-Baroux J, Siegler A. Diagnosis and treatment of intra- uterine adhesions by microhysteroscopy. Fertil Steril. 1983;39:321–6.
24. Valle RF, Sciarra JJ. Intrauterine adhesions: hysteroscopic diagnosis, classification, treatment, and reproductive outcome. Am J Obstet Gynecol. 1988;158:1459–70.
25. The American Fertility Society classifications of adnexal adhesions, distal tubal occlusion, tubal occlusion secondary to tubal ligation, tubal pregnancies, mullerian anomalies and intrauterine adhesions. Fertil Steril. 1988;49:944–55.
26. Polishuk WZ, Siew FP, Gordon R, Lebenshart P. Vascular changes in traumatic amenorrhea and hypomenorrhea. Int J Fertil. 1977;22:189–92.
27. Soares SR, Barbosa dos Reis MM, Camargos AF. Diagnostic accuracy of sonohysterography, transvaginal sonography, and hysterosalpingography in patients with uterine cavity diseases. Fertil Steril. 2000;73:406–11.
28. Sylvestre C, Child TJ, Tulandi T, Tan SL. A prospective study to evaluate the efficacy of two- and three-dimensional sonohysterography in women with intrauterine lesions. Fertil Steril. 2003;79:1222–5.
29. Salle B, Gaucherand P, de Saint Hilaire P, Rudigoz RC. Transvaginal sonohysterographic evaluation of intrauterine adhesions. J Clin Ultrasound. 1999;27:131–4.
30. Seshadri S, El-Toukhy T, Douiri A, Jayaprakasan K, Khalaf Y. Diagnostic accuracy of saline infusion sonography in the evaluation of uterine cavity abnormalities prior to assisted reproductive techniques: a systematic review and meta-analyses. Hum Reprod Update. 2015;21(2):262–74.
31. Yang JH, Chen CD, Chen SU, Yang YS, Chen MJ. The influence of the location and extent of intrauterine adhesions on recurrence after hysteroscopic adhesiolysis. BJOG. 2016;123(4):618–23.
32. Letterie GS, Haggerty MF. MRI: Magnetic resonance imaging of intrauterine synechiae. Gynecol Obstet Invest. 1994;37(1):66–8.
33. Bacelar AC, Wilcock D, Powell M, Worthington BS. The value of MRI in the assessment of traumatic intra-uterine adhesions (Asherman's syndrome). Clin Radiol. 1995;50:80–3.
34. Raziel A, Arieli S, Bukovsky I, Caspi E, Golan A. Investigation of the uterine cavity in recurrent aborters. Fertil Steril. 1994;62(5):1080–2.
35. Asimakopulos N. Traumatic intrauterine adhesions. (the fritsch-asherman syndrome). Can Med Assoc J. 1965;93:298–302.
36. Louros NC, Danezis JM, Pontifix G. Use of intrauterine devices in the treatment of intrauterine adhesions. Fertil Steril. 1968;19(4):509–28.
37. Klein SM, García CR. Asherman's syndrome: a critique and current review. Fertil Steril. 1973;24(9):722–35.
38. Levine RU, Neuwirth RS. Simultaneous laparoscopy and hysteroscopy for intrauterine adhesions. Obstet Gynecol. 1973;42(3):441–5.
39. March CM, Israel R, March AD. Hysteroscopic management of intrauterine adhesions. Am J Obstet Gynecol. 1978;130(6):653–7.
40. Sciarra JJ, Valle RF. Hysteroscopy: a clinical experience with 320 patients. Am J Obstet Gynecol. 1977;127(4):340–8.
41. Sanfilippo JS, Fitzgerald MR, Badawy SZ, Nussbaum ML, Yussman MA. Asherman's syndrome. A comparison of therapeutic methods. J Reprod Med. 1982;27(6):328–30.
42. Lancet M, Mass N. Concomitant hysteroscopy and hysterography in Asherman's syndrome. Int J Fertil. 1981;26(4):267–72.
43. Fernandez H, Peyrelevade S, Legendre G, Faivre E, Deffieux X, Nazac A. Total adhesions treated by hysteroscopy: must we stop at two procedures? Fertil Steril. 2012;98(4):980–5.
44. Xiao S, Wan Y, Xue M, Zeng X, Xiao F, Xu D, Yang X, Zhang P, Sheng W, Xu J, Zhou S. Etiology, treatment, and reproductive prognosis of women with moderate-to-severe intrauterine adhesions. Int J Gynaecol Obstet. 2014;125(2):121–4.

45. Wortman M, Daggett A, Ball C. Operative hysteroscopy in an office-based surgical setting: review of patient safety and satisfaction in 414 cases. J Minim Invasive Gynecol. 2013;20(1):56–63.
46. Chervenak FA, Neuwirth RS. Hysteroscopic resection of the uterine septum. Am J Obstet Gynecol. 1981;141(3):351.
47. Duffy S, Reid PC, Sharp F. In-vivo studies of uterine electrosurgery. Br J Obstet Gynaecol. 1992;99:579–82.
48. Zikopoulos KA, Kolibianakis EM, Platteau P, de Munck L, Tournaye H, Devroey P, Camus M. Live delivery rates in subfertile women with Asherman's syndrome after hysteroscopic adhesiolysis using the resectoscope or the Versapoint system. Reprod Biomed Online. 2004;8:720–5.
49. Newton JR, MacKenzie WE, Emens MJ, Jordan JA. Division of uterine adhesions (Asherman's syndrome) with the Nd-YAG laser. Br J Obstet Gynaecol. 1989;96:102–4.
50. Chapman R, Chapman K. The value of two stage laser treatment for severe Asherman's syndrome. Br J Obstet Gynaecol. 1996;103:1256–8.
51. Nappi L, Pontis A, Sorrentino F, Greco P, Angioni S. Hysteroscopic metroplasty for the septate uterus with diode laser: a pilot study. Eur J Obstet Gynecol Reprod Biol. 2016;206:32–5.
52. Lo KW, Yuen PM. Hysteroscopic metroplasty under laparoscopic ultrasound guidance. Acta Obstet Gynecol Scand. 1998;77(5):580–1.
53. McComb PF, Wagner BL. Simplified therapy for Asherman's syndrome. Fertil Steril. 1997;68(6):1047–50.
54. Berman JM. Intrauterine adhesions. Semin Reprod Med. 2008;26(4):349–55.
55. Coccia ME, Becattini C, Bracco GL, Bargelli G, Scarselli G. Intraoperative ultrasound guidance for operative hysteroscopy. A prospective study. J Reprod Med. 2000;45(5):413–8.
56. Kresowik JD, Syrop CH, Van Voorhis BJ, Ryan GL. Ultrasound is the optimal choice for guidance in difficult hysteroscopy. Ultrasound Obstet Gynecol. 2012;39(6):715–8.
57. Vigoureux S, Fernandez H, Capmas P, Levaillant JM, Legendre G. Assessment of abdominal ultrasound guidance in hysteroscopic metroplasty. J Minim Invasive Gynecol. 2016;23(1):78–83.
58. Hayasaka S, Murakami T, Arai M, Ugajin T, Nabeshima H, Yuki H, Terada Y, Yaegashi N. J Gynecol Surg. 2009;25(4):147–52.
59. Thomson AJ, Abbott JA, Kingston A, Lenart M, Vancaillie TG. Fluoroscopically guided synechiolysis for patients with Asherman's syndrome: menstrual and fertility outcomes. Fertil Steril. 2007;87(2):405–10.
60. Protopapas A, Shushan A, Magos A. Myometrial scoring: a new technique for the management of severe Asherman's syndrome. Fertil Steril. 1998;69:860–4.
61. Pabuccu R, Onalan G, Kaya C, Selam B, Ceyhan T, Ornek T, Kuzudisli E. Efficiency and pregnancy outcome of serial intrauterine device-guided hysteroscopic adhesiolysis of intrauterine synechiae. Fertil Steril. 2008;90(5):1973–7.
62. Agostini A, Cravello L, Desbrière R, Maisonneuve AS, Roger V, Blanc B. Hemorrhage risk during operative hysteroscopy. Acta Obstet Gynecol Scand. 2002;81(9):878–81.
63. Pasini A, Belloni C. Intraoperative complications of 697 consecutive operative hysteroscopies. Minerva Ginecol. 2001;53(1):13–20.
64. Scoccia B, Demir H, Elter K, Scommegna A. Successful medical management of post-hysteroscopic metroplasty bleeding with intravenous estrogen therapy: a report of two cases and review of the literature. J Minim Invasive Gynecol. 2009;16(5):639–42.
65. Agostini A, Cravello L, Bretelle F, Shojai R, Roger V, Blanc B. Risk of uterine perforation during hysteroscopic surgery. J Am Assoc Gynecol Laparosc. 2002;9(3):264–7.
66. Xia EL, Duan H, Zhang J, Chen F, Wang SM, Zhang PJ, Yu D, Zheng J, Huang XW. Analysis of 16 cases of uterine perforation during hysteroscopic electro-surgeries. Zhonghua Fu Chan Ke Za Zhi. 2003;38(5):280–3.
67. Yang BJ, Feng LM. Symptomatic hyponatremia and hyperglycemia complicating hysteroscopic resection of intrauterine adhesion: a case report. Chin Med J (Engl). 2012;125(8):1508–10.

68. Yu D, Li TC, Xia E, Huang X, Liu Y, Peng X. Factors affecting reproductive outcome of hysteroscopic adhesiolysis for Asherman's syndrome. Fertil Steril. 2008;89(3):715–22.

69. Sentilhes L, Sergent F, Roman H, Verspyck E, Marpeau L. Late complications of operative hysteroscopy: predicting patients at risk of uterine rupture during subsequent pregnancy. Eur J Obstet Gynecol Reprod Biol. 2005;120(2):134–8.

70. Robinson JK, Colimon LM, Isaacson KB. Postoperative adhesiolysis therapy for intrauterine adhesions (Asherman's syndrome). Fertil Steril. 2008;90(2):409–14.

71. de Rozada IB, Rozada H, Remedio MR, Sica-Blanco Y. IUD in the treatment of uterine synechiae. Obstet Gynecol. 1968;32(3):387–90.

72. Polishuk WZ, Weinstein D. The Soichet intrauterine device in the treatment of intrauterine adhesions. Acta Eur Fertil. 1976;7(3):215–8.

73. Ismajovich B, Lidor A, Confino E, David MP. Treatment of minimal and moderate intrauterine adhesions (Asherman's syndrome). J Reprod Med. 1985;30(10):769–72.

74. Zwinger A, Schönfeld V, Mares J, Valenta M. The use of an intra-uterine contraceptive pessary in the treatment of women infertile due to uterine synechiae. Zentralbl Gynakol. 1969;91(2):63–7.

75. Maneschi M, Vegna G, Mezzatesta M. Use of Lippes Loop in the treatment of post-traumatic uterine adhesions. Minerva Ginecol. 1974;26(11):633–40.

76. Massouras HG, Coutifaris B, Kalogirou D. Management of uterine adhesions with 'Massouras Duck's Foot' and 'Butterfly' IUDs. Contracept Deliv Syst. 1982;3(1):25–38.

77. Salma U, Xue M, Sayed ASM, Xu D. Efficacy of intrauterine device in the treatment of intrauterine adhesions. Biomed Res Int. 2014;2014:589296., 15 pages. https://doi.org/10.1155/2014/589296.

78. March CM. Intrauterine adhesions. Obstet Gynecol Clin North Am. 1995;22:491–505.

79. Vercellini P, Fedele L, Arcaini L, Rognoni MT, Candiani GB. Value of intrauterine device insertion and estrogen administration after hysteroscopic metroplasty. J Reprod Med. 1989;34(7):447–50.

80. Pabuccu R, Atay V, Orhon E, et al. Hysteroscopic treatment of intrauterine adhesions is safe and effective in the restoration of normal menstruation and fertility. Fertil Steril. 1997;68:1141–3.

81. Tonguc EA, Var T, Yilmaz N, Batioglu S. Intrauterine device or estrogen treatment after hysteroscopic uterine septum resection. Int J Gynaecol Obstet. 2010;109(3):226–9.

82. Lin XN, Zhou F, Wei ML, Yang Y, Li Y, Li TC, Zhang SY. Randomized, controlled trial comparing the efficacy of intrauterine balloon and intrauterine contraceptive device in the prevention of adhesion reformation after hysteroscopic adhesiolysis. Fertil Steril. 2015;104(1):235–40.

83. Goorah B, Tulandi T. Uterine rupture resulting from the pressure of an intrauterine balloon. J Obstet Gynaecol Can. 2009;31(7):649–51.

84. Gupta S, Talaulikar VS, Onwude J, Manyonda I. A pilot study of Foley's catheter balloon for prevention of intrauterine adhesions following breach of uterine cavity in complex myoma surgery. Arch Gynecol Obstet. 2013;288(4):829–32.

85. Lin X, Wei M, Li TC, Huang Q, Huang D, Zhou F, Zhang S. A comparison of intrauterine balloon, intrauterine contraceptive device and hyaluronic acid gel in the prevention of adhesion reformation following hysteroscopic surgery for Asherman syndrome: a cohort study. Eur J Obstet Gynecol Reprod Biol. 2013;170(2):512–6.

86. Amer MI, El Nadim A, Hassanein K. The role of intrauterine balloon after operative hysteroscopy in the prevention of intrauterine adhesion: a prospective controlled study. MEFS J. 2005;10:125–9.

87. Orhue AA, Aziken ME, Igbefoh JO. A comparison of two adjunctive treatments for intrauterine adhesions following lysis. Int J Gynaecol Obstet. 2003;82(1):49–56.

88. Yu X, Yuhan L, Dongmei S, Enlan X, Tinchiu L. The incidence of post-operative adhesion following transection of uterine septum: a cohort study comparing three different adjuvant therapies. Eur J Obstet Gynecol Reprod Biol. 2016;2016:1–4.

89. Amer MI, Abd-El-Maeboud KH. Amnion graft following hysteroscopic lysis of intrauterine adhesions. J Obstet Gynaecol Res. 2006;32:559–66.
90. Amer MI, Abd-El-Maeboud KH, Abdelfatah I, Salama FA, Abdallah AS. Human amnion as a temporary biologic barrier after hysteroscopic lysis of severe intrauterine adhesions: pilot study. J Minim Invasive Gynecol. 2010;17(5):605–11.
91. Acunzo G, Guida M, Pellicano M, Tommaselli GA, Di Spiezio Sardo A, Bifulco G, Cirillo D, Taylor A, Nappi C. Effectiveness of auto-cross-linked hyaluronic acid gel in the prevention of intrauterine adhesions after hysteroscopic adhesiolysis: a prospective, randomized, controlled study. Hum Reprod. 2003;18(9):1918–21.
92. Kim T, Ahn KH, Choi DS, Hwang KJ, Lee BI, Jung MH, Kim JW, Kim JH, Cha SH, Lee KH, Lee KS, Oh ST, Cho CH, Rhee JH. A randomized, multi-center, clinical trial to assess the efficacy and safety of alginate carboxymethylcellulose hyaluronic acid compared to carboxymethylcellulose hyaluronic acid to prevent postoperative intrauterine adhesion. J Minim Invasive Gynecol. 2012;19(6):731–6.
93. Tsapanos VS, Stathopoulou LP, Papathanassopoulou VS, Tzingounis VA. The role of Seprafilm bioresorbable membrane in the prevention and therapy of endometrial synechiae. J Biomed Mater Res. 2002;63(1):10–4.
94. Bosteels J, Weyers S, Mol BW, D'Hooghe T. Anti-adhesion barrier gels following operative hysteroscopy for treating female infertility: a systematic review and meta-analysis. Gynecol Surg. 2014;11:113–27.
95. Comninos AC, Zourlas PA. Treatment of uterine adhesions (Asherman's syndrome). Am J Obstet Gynecol. 1969;105(6):862–8.
96. Asch RH, Zuo WL, Garcia M, Ramzy I, Laufe L, Rojas FP. Intrauterine release of oestriol in castrated rhesus monkeys induces local but not peripheral oestrogenic effects: a possible approach for the treatment and prevention of Asherman's syndrome. Hum Reprod. 1991;6(10):1373–8.
97. Farhi J, Bar-Hava I, Homburg R, Dicker D, Ben-Rafael Z. Induced regeneration of endometrium following curettage for abortion: a comparative study. Hum Reprod. 1993;8(7):1143–4.
98. Dawood A, Al-Talib A, Tulandi T. Predisposing factors and treatment outcome of different stages of intra-uterine adhesions. J Obstet Gynaecol Can. 2010;32:767–70.
99. Roy KK, Negi N, Subbaiah M, Kumar S, Sharma JB, Singh N. Effectiveness of estrogen in the prevention of intrauterine adhesions after hysteroscopic septal resection: a prospective, randomized study. J Obstet Gynaecol Res. 2014;40(4):1085–8.
100. Healy MW, Schexnayder B, Connell MT, Terry N, DeCherney AH, Csokmay JM, Yauger BJ, Hill MJ. Intrauterine adhesion prevention after hysteroscopy: a systematic review and meta-analysis. Am J Obstet Gynecol. 2016;215(3):267–75.
101. Bosteels J, Weyers S, Kasius J, Broekmans FJ, Mol BW, D'Hooghe TM. Anti-adhesion therapy following operative hysteroscopy for treatment of female subfertility. Cochrane Database Syst Rev. 2015;11:CD011110.
102. Pace S, Stentella P, Catania R, Palazzetti PL, Frega A. Endoscopic treat- ment of intrauterine adhesions. Clin Exp Obstet Gynecol. 2003;30:26–8.
103. Katz Z, Ben-Arie A, Lurie S, Manor M, Insler V. Reproductive outcome following hysteroscopic adhesiolysis in Asherman's syndrome. Int J Fertil Menopausal Stud. 1996;41:462–5.
104. March CM. Management of Asherman's syndrome. Reprod Biomed Online. 2011;23(1):63–76.
105. Bhandari S, Bhave P, Ganguly I, Baxi A, Agarwal P. Reproductive outcome of patients with Asherman's syndrome: a SAIMS experience. J Reprod Infertil. 2015;16(4):229–35.
106. Chen L, Zhang H, Wang Q, Xie F, Gao S, Song Y, Dong J, Feng H, Xie K, Sui L. Reproductive outcomes in patients with intrauterine adhesions following hysteroscopic adhesiolysis: experience from the largest women's hospital in China. J Minim Invasive Gynecol. 2017;24(2):299–304.

Role of Hysteroscopy in ART

9

Parag Hitnalikar

9.1 Introduction

Although ART has been a boon for infertile couples, the failure rate is still more than the success rate. In order to increase the take-home baby rate, continuous scientific efforts are being put at various stages of IVF cycle. But still the understanding of all the factors leading to failure is limited.

To get optimum results, factors that are closely related to the outcome need to be defined. Factors that stand out are quality of embryo, condition and receptivity of the uterus, and technical efficiency of embryologist and clinician. In this chapter, we will be focusing mainly on the intrauterine environment and methods to diagnose and correct intrauterine pathologies. In a study by Prevedourakis et al., it has been found that as many as 50% of infertile females have some or the other uterine pathology [1]. The intrauterine pathologies which are significantly associated with negative outcome are endometrial polyp, intrauterine adhesions, uterine septum, leiomyoma, endometritis, and endometrial hyperplasia [2]. Optimizing the chances of success in the very first IVF cycle can lead to overall reduction in cost to achieve pregnancy. It is therefore imperative to diagnose any intrauterine pathology before IVF cycle. Of the various methods available for assessment of uterine cavity, hysteroscopy has come out as a significantly better modality.

9.2 Assessment of Uterine Cavity

The assessment of uterine cavity can be done by transvaginal sonography (TVS), saline infusion sonography (SIS), hysterosalpingography (HSG), and hysteroscopy. The simplest and most cost-effective way to diagnose uterine pathology is by

P. Hitnalikar, MD (OBGY), FNB (Reprod Med)
Orion Hospital, Pune, Maharashtra, India

Ruby Hall Clinic, Pune, Maharashtra, India

© Springer Nature Singapore Pte Ltd. 2018
S. Jain, D. B. Inamdar (eds.), *Manual of Fertility Enhancing Hysteroscopy*,
https://doi.org/10.1007/978-981-10-8028-9_9

TVS. We can study the myometrium, endometrial lining and blood flow, uterine contour, and volumetric assessment with high accuracy. But some intrauterine pathologies such as endometritis or intrauterine synechiae cannot be ruled out by TVS [3]. TVS can diagnose the intrauterine pathologies with sensitivity of 84–100% and specificity of 96.3–98% [4]. To improve on plain TVS, saline infusion sonography was introduced which is superior to TVS in studying intrauterine pathologies, uterine contour, and endometrial assessment. HSG can also be used to assess the uterine cavity, but it is associated with significant pain, allergic reactions to contrast media, and vasovagal shock due to cervical stimulation. Moreover we are likely to miss out on a significant number of intrauterine pathologies as the false-positive rate of HSG is 15.6% and false-negative rate is 34.4% [5].

Hysteroscopy has proven time and again to be a gold standard for uterine assessment [6, 7]. Most of the intrauterine pathologies can be accurately diagnosed by hysteroscopy; moreover, many of the pathologies can be treated simultaneously. Hysteroscopy has significantly improved the assessment of endometrial pathologies over TVS and HSG. Even when other modalities have shown no significant pathology, hysteroscopy has detected abnormalities in 18–50% of patients undergoing IVF [8].

Hysteroscopy can be employed in the ART in three conditions:

(a) In those patients who are showing abnormality on HSG or SIS
(b) Repeated IVF failures
(c) Routinely before all IVF cycles

9.3   Procedure

Traditionally hysteroscopy is performed as indoor procedure, in operation theater under sedatives or anesthesia. Older hysteroscopes were having larger diameters requiring cervical dilatation and anesthesia to avoid pain and discomfort. But recently, evolution of small-caliber hysteroscopes and use of vaginoscopic approach, hysteroscopy can be performed without the need of anesthesia with excellent patient compliance. Vaginoscopic approach also rules out the need for premedication, thereby performing the procedure faster with very rare complications [9]. With advancement of technology, now various miniaturized hysteroscopes, hand instruments, and electrical sources are rendering treatment of various uterine pathologies in office settings. A review done by De Spizo Sardo et al. [10] conclusively demonstrated that various intrauterine pathologies such as endometrial polyps, intrauterine adhesions, anatomical disorders, biopsies, and small myomas can be operated safely and successfully without need of cervical dilatation or anesthesia.

A variety of hysteroscopes are available with diameter ranging from 2.9 to 5 mm using which office hysteroscopy can be done before ART. Recent evidence suggests that if the hysteroscopy done in 6 months preceding the IVF cycle, it is more beneficial. Hysteroscopy should be done in follicular phase of the cycle to get a better assessment of uterine cavity. The findings such as direction of internal os, the presence of any fibrotic bands in the lower uterine tract, cervical and uterocervical lengths, and direction of uterine cavity should be noted. In case of suspicion, endometrial sampling for infection should be taken. Patients are given analgesics and antispasmodics when required after the procedure.

9.4   Prevalence

Prevalence of unsuspected intrauterine pathologies has been reported to be between 20% and 45% [8, 11–14]. In a study by Rana Karayalcin et al., [15] 2500 infertile females were subjected for diagnostic hysteroscopy before IVF cycle prospectively. The study was performed in a single IVF center in office setting. Out of the study population of consecutive infertile patients, 22.9% had some or the other uterine pathology, and 77.1% patients had normal uterus. The most common uterine pathology was endometrial polyp in 192 (7.7%) patients followed by Mullerian anomalies mainly uterine septum in 130 (5.2%) subjects. The other significant findings were myoma (3.8%), polypoid endometrium (1.2%), and intrauterine adhesions (1.1%). This study shows that in unsuspected population, significant number of infertile women have uterine findings which can hamper the positive outcome in IVF cycle. The findings of the study are shown in Table 9.1 [15].

Many of the studies done to measure prevalence were done with prior evaluation by either with TVS or HSG. Still there is quite high number of cases where some intrauterine pathology is found. It prompts us to evaluate all the uterine cavities by hysteroscopy before ART. In the following few paragraphs, we will study the most common pathologies and proposed mechanisms of pathogenesis.

Table 9.1 Findings of 2500 hysteroscopies included in study [15]

Finding	Number	Percentage
Normal	1927	77.1
Abnormal	573	22.9
Endometrial polyp	192	7.7
Mullerian anomalies (septum)	130	5.2
Myoma	96	3.8
Mullerian anomalies (bicornuate uterus)	28	1.1
Polypoid endometrium	31	1.2
Adhesions	27	1.1
Endometrial hyperplasia	22	0.9
T-shaped uterus	18	0.7
Endometritis	13	0.5
Cervical polyps	13	0.5
Cervical stenosis	3	0.1

Source: "Results of 2500 office-based diagnostic hysteroscopies before IVF," by Karayalcin et al., 2010, Reproductive BioMedicine Online; 20:689–93. Copyright 2010. Reproduced with permission from Elsevier

9.5   Common Pathologies of Concern for Successful ART Cycle

9.5.1   Leiomyoma

By far the most common benign tumors of uterine origin in women of reproductive age group are uterine leiomyoma. The prevalence is reported to be as high as 70–80% in female population by the age of 50 years [16]. Leiomyomas are found in 5–10% of females suffering from infertility, and it is the only detectable pathology in 1–2.4% of the infertile females. There are various mechanisms by which leiomyoma can interfere with fertility. The most common mechanism is distortion of endometrial cavity and mechanical obstruction to either cervix hampering sperm transport or osteal openings affecting embryo movement [17]. Not only in natural cycles but myomas can significantly reduce success rate in ART cycles [18]. Myomectomy has been shown to significantly improve pregnancy rates in otherwise unexplained infertility, and pregnancy rate of 40–60% was achieved at the end of 2 years [19]. At the molecular level, myomas affect overlying endometrium and have been shown to significantly hamper implantation rate, although the data is limited in support of this hypothesis [20, 21]. During the time of implantation, expression of HOXA 10, HOXA 11, and BTEB 1 genes, which are important for implantation, was studied, and it was found to be significantly low in uteri having submucous leiomyoma as compared to normal uteri [20, 21]. It was also found that expression of HOXA 10 gene was affected not only in the overlying endometrium but whole of the endometrial tissue [21]. This suggests that apart from mechanical interference and focal affection, leiomyomas affect globally thus reducing overall implantation rate. Recent Cochrane review also suggests that large benefit with the hysteroscopic removal of submucous fibroids for improving the chance of clinical pregnancy in women with otherwise unexplained subfertility cannot be excluded [22] (Fig. 9.1).

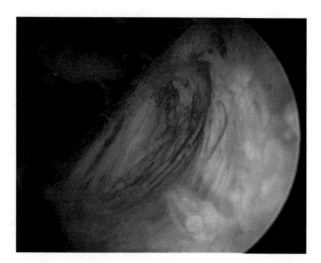

Fig. 9.1 Resection of intramural fibroid

9.5.2   Endometrial Polyp

Endometrial polyps are benign localized overgrowths of the endometrium. It is not yet fully understood how the polyp interferes with pregnancy, but few mechanisms proposed are interference with sperm transport, interference with embryo transport, or abnormal expression of markers of implantation. Low expression of certain markers such as IGFBP-1 and osteopontin has been found in uterine flushings of mid-luteal phase endometrium in females with endometrial polyp [23]. When polypectomy was performed, levels of the same markers have been found to be significantly increased [23]. For successful implantation, normal expression of progesterone receptors is required. In patients with uterine polyp, abnormal expression of progesterone receptors was found because of progesterone resistance [24]. The prevalence of endometrial polyp on hysteroscopy in reproductive age group with unexplained infertility is 16–26%, but in infertile population with endometriosis, the same rate is as high as 46% [25, 26]. Very few studies have been conducted to examine the effect of polyp on fertility. Only one randomized study has shown a significant improvement in pregnancy rate in IUI cycles following polypectomy (63% vs. 28%) [27]. Three other nonrandomized trials comparing spontaneous pregnancy rates after polypectomy also suggested significant improvement in pregnancy rate [28]. In IVF cycles, the effect of endometrial polyp is not very clear. Endometrial polyp <2 cm in size has limited effect on the IVF outcome, but further studies are required to assess the impact of size, number, and location of endometrial polyps on IVF success [29, 30] (Figs. 9.2, 9.3, and 9.4).

9.5.3   Endometritis

Endometrial infection by variety of pathogens has been implicated in infertility and implantation failure because of various inflammatory products secreted by

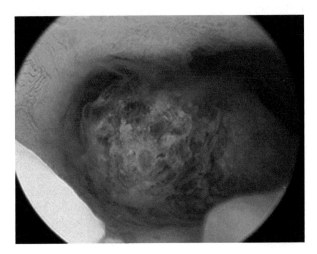

Fig. 9.2 Endometrial polyp

Fig. 9.3 Resection of
endometrial polyp by
scissor

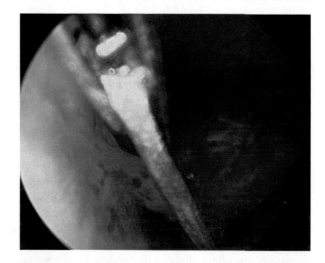

Fig. 9.4 Polypoidal
endometrium

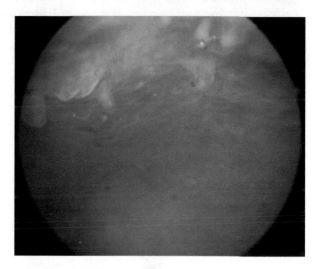

microbes [31]. The implantation rate and clinical pregnancy rates have been lower
in females with chronic endometritis (8% and 11%) as compared to females with
negative endometrial biopsies (31% and 58%) [32]. When endometrial biopsy
was taken in patients during pre-IVF hysteroscopy, acute endometritis was found
in 15% of nonselected patients, where as it was as high as 42% in cases of repeated
implantation failure [33]. When suitable antibiotic therapy was given in those
patients with endometritis, significant improvement in IVF success was observed
in subsequent cycle.

Endometritis can be acute or chronic. Acute endometritis is generally caused by
bacteria and is transient in nature. It is not associated with long-standing infertility.
It responds well to antibiotic therapy. Chronic endometritis can be caused by

Fig. 9.5 Tubercular
endometrium

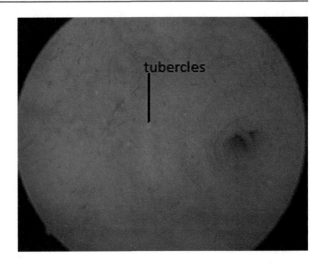

bacteria, viruses, or parasites. It is associated with chronic inflammatory reaction in endometrium and may be a cause of prolonged infertility. In developing countries, tuberculosis is a common and significant cause of pelvic inflammatory diseases and is associated with significantly reduced fertility. It affects the females of reproductive age groups (20–40 years), and it can remain silent for quite a long time till it is diagnosed in infertility workup [34]. It is generally secondary to infection elsewhere in the body. Primary target of genital infection is fallopian tubes which are involved in almost all cases followed by endometrium and ovaries. It causes significant destruction of tubal and endometrial linings and is associated with reduced success rate in IVF cycles (Fig. 9.5).

9.5.4   Intrauterine Adhesions

Intrauterine adhesions are a significant cause of repeated implantation failure. It occurs more commonly after pelvic inflammatory disease, vigorous curetting of endometrial cavity, or postpartum sepsis. Adhesions can be flimsy and superficial which do not have significant effect on fertility. But thick and fibrotic adhesions are associated with infertility and repeated implantation failure. Thick adhesions cause fibrosis and scarring of adjoining area and also reduce endometrial blood flow. Adhesion formation can be prevented by the use of high-dose estradiol or mechanical distention of endometrial cavity after surgery. Newer modalities such as the use of anti-adhesive barriers are also showing promising results for prevention of adhesion formation. Pre-IVF hysteroscopy facilitates diagnosis as well as treatment of intrauterine adhesions which are difficult to pick up on any other modality. Studies have shown that adhesiolysis in patient with intrauterine adhesions significantly improves IVF outcome [35]. Patient should also be counseled regarding possibility of pregnancy complications such as placenta accreta.

9.5.5 Uterine Septum

Uterine septum is a Mullerian anomaly presenting as centrally placed fibromuscular overgrowth in endometrial cavity. It may vary in extent from partial to complete septum and is associated with distortion of the uterine cavity and reduction in intra-uterine space. The endometrial development and vascularity are generally poor in the overlying endometrium. It is most commonly associated with recurrent abortions. Treatment of uterine septum at the time of diagnosis is associated with significant improvement in live birth, and it can also be considered as the first-line treatment in patient undergoing infertility treatment [36]. Resection of uterine septum by hysteroscopy is associated with significant improvement in fecundity in patients with unexplained infertility [37]. No randomized studies are available to compare outcome of hysteroscopic resection in patients undergoing IVF cycles; hence, the impact of hysteroscopic resection is till inconclusive, and further studies are required [38].

9.6 Role of Hysteroscopy in ART

In search of improving the final outcome of IVF cycles, many attempts are made in terms of improving the implantation rates. One of the basic prerequisite for good implantation is having a receptive uterine cavity. Studies were conducted to assess the uterine cavity by hysteroscopy before the ART cycle. These studies mainly can be divided in answering two important questions as follows.

9.6.1 Is Hysteroscopy Helpful in Previous Failed IVF Cycle?

Studies performed on patients with previous one or more failed IVF cycles have conclusively proven that pre-IVF hysteroscopy improves the clinical outcome in these patients [12, 14, 39, 40].

Demirol et al. [12] conducted a study to evaluate the effect of office hysteroscopy in patients with repeated implantation failures. The study included 421 patients who had previous two or more failed IVF cycles and divided in two groups. Group I ($n = 211$) included patients who did not undergo pre-IVF hysteroscopy, and group II included patients who underwent hysteroscopy. Group II was further divided in IIa and IIb comprising of patients who had no findings on hysteroscopy and patients having abnormal findings on hysteroscopy, respectively. Group IIb was simultaneously treated in the same setting. Clinical pregnancy rates in groups I, IIa, and IIb were 21.6%, 32.5%, and 30.4%, respectively. There was significant difference in groups I and II, which proved that there was improvement in IVF outcome if the patients underwent hysteroscopy before IVF. More importantly there was no significant difference in the outcome of patients who had normal and abnormal findings on hysteroscopy, which prompts to benefits of hysteroscopy other than correction of pathology. Hence they concluded that patients with repeated implantation failure should undergo pre-IVF hysteroscopy.

Evidence also suggest that in patients with previous two or more failed IVF attempts, controlled endometrial injury during day 7 of previous cycle up to day 7 of cycle in which ET is performed improves success rate. Moreover no effect on miscarriage, bleeding, or multiple pregnancy rates has been observed because of endometrial injury [41].

9.6.2 Is Hysteroscopy Helpful in First IVF Cycle?

Although studies are done on outcome of hysteroscopy in repeated IVF failures, effect of hysteroscopy before first IVF cycle is not studied systematically. In a review by Pundir et al. [42], only one randomized and five nonrandomized studies were suitable for inclusion. The prevalence of intrauterine pathologies was found to be as high as 50%. They concluded that if hysteroscopy was performed before IVF cycle in patients irrespective of clinical suspicion, improvement in IVF outcome was possible. They also concluded that further randomized studies are necessary to evaluate effect of hysteroscopy on IVF success rate.

Even in asymptomatic patients, intrauterine pathologies such as endometrial polyp, septum, leiomyoma, and intrauterine adhesions are found in significant numbers. All these intrauterine pathologies are likely to result in adverse IVF outcome. Correction and treatment of these pathologies will have impact on the intrauterine environment and implantation potential of the endometrium. Pre-IVF hysteroscopy can have effects on the IVF outcome not only by correction of the existing pathologies but in other ways that are not clearly understood. In few studies it was found that dilatation of cervix increases ease of doing embryo transfer, thereby reducing trauma to endometrium and more accurate placement of embryos. Stimulation of endometrium has been considered as the probable factors increasing IVF success rate by improving implantation potential [43–45]. In a study by Doldi et al. [8], they intentionally performed endometrial biopsy after hysteroscopy and found that pregnancy rate was improved in patient group which underwent endometrial biopsy.

In order to improve implantation rate, endometrial scratching has gained a lot of popularity. The underlying mechanism through which endometrial injury improves implantation is still unclear. There are three main supposed theories. First is through inducing decidualization of endometrium, which might improve the implantation [46]. Second is that the process of healing after endometrial injury involves an inflammatory reaction mediated with cytokines, interleukins, growth factors, macrophages, and dendritic cells, which are beneficial to embryo implantation [46–48]. The third is that endometrial injury in previous cycle leads to better synchronicity between endometrium and transferred embryos through retarding endometrial maturation [46].

Implantation requires a synchrony of expression of various endometrial factors. In ERA, study of 238 genes responsible for expression of factors required at different stages of implantation is done. Data is collected about expression of these genes and used for calculating personalized window of implantation. Each patient has a different receptivity status of the endometrium, and synchronization of embryo transfer with endometrial receptivity improves the chances of successful implantation [49]. ERA is more accurate as compared to endometrial histology. It is also more reproducible as the receptivity status of the endometrium was same when the test was performed after 29–40 months of the first test [50].

9.7   Recent Advances of Hysteroscopy in ART

9.7.1   Hysteroscopic-Guided Embryo Transfer

One of the rate limiting steps of IVF success is proper embryo transfer. Out of the many ways suggested to improve embryo transfer, hysteroscopic-guided embryo transfer is one with logical appeal. In this procedure, small-caliber hysteroscope is used to visualize the cervix first. Either CO_2 or nitrous oxide gas is used to distend uterine cavity. Outer catheter is attached to the hysteroscope, and catheter is inserted in the endometrial cavity under vision which is followed by embryo placement by inner catheter.

The possible benefits by this technique are circumventing negotiation difficulty at the internal os, fewer chances of trauma, and less chances of ectopic pregnancy. In some studies, successful pregnancies along with reduced risk of ectopic pregnancies, increased success rate has been reported [51], but in a systematic review by Abu Setta et al., they concluded that there is no strong evidence that hysteroscopic embryo (cleavage or blastocyst) transfer is more beneficial than either routine clinical touch or ultrasound-guided embryo transfer [52]. This novel technique requires more studies to establish its real usefulness.

9.7.2   Hysteroscopic Tubal Occlusion

The effect of hydrosalphinges on IVF has been amply documented, and it has been shown to significantly decrease implantation and clinical pregnancy rate [53]. Laparoscopic tubal occlusion has been a well-established approach to avoid the negative effects of hydrosalphinges on IVF outcome. Alternatively tubal occlusion can also be achieved by hysteroscopic methods. This can be done by using ball cautery or special devices such as Essure (Bayer, USA).

Darwish and El Saman [54] conducted a study which compares the IVF outcome in patients who underwent hysteroscopic tubal occlusion versus laparoscopic tubal occlusion in functionless hydrosalpinx before IVF cycle. They used roller ball electrode of resectoscope to occlude the tubal ostia hysteroscopically. They concluded that hysteroscopic tubal occlusion produces similar results as compared to laparoscopic tubal occlusion, and it also has got an added advantage of inspection of endometrial cavity.

In those patients, in which laparoscopy is difficult or contraindicated, Essure microinsert can be placed in the tubal ostia by hysteroscopic route. The procedure is described in detail in a separate chapter.

9.7.3 Cervical Refashioning

There is a certain subgroup of failed IVF cycles due to extremely difficult embryo transfer. Traumatic ET poses a significant difficulty in these patients, and many techniques were suggested to overcome this problem with very little success. Even cervical dilatation at the time of OPU or in previous cycle has not met with significant success in these patients [55].

Noyes in 1999 suggested a surgical approach for this cervical stenosis by excising excess of cervical tissue hysteroscopically by resectoscope. This procedure creates a smooth cervical canal which facilitates easy embryo transfer [56]. Recently versapoint twizzle is used to shave cervical tissue which is less traumatic and requires minimum dilatation because of small caliber of instrument. Linear incisions are made in cervical canal, thereby releasing fibrotic tissue which is followed by cervical dilatation to stretch the fibrous tissue further. It has been shown to significantly improve the ease of doing embryo transfers in subsequent cycles [57].

Conclusion

Lot of efforts has been put to study the uterine cavity before ART cycle in order to improve the success rate. Out of all the available modalities available for evaluation of uterine cavity, hysteroscopy is considered as gold standard. Many pathological conditions of endometrium including some subtle ones can hamper implantation of embryos and produce adverse ART outcome. Employing hysteroscopy in cases of recurrent ART failures as well as routinely before all ART cycles is likely to improve the success rate of the cycle.

References

1. Prevedourakis C, Loutradis D, Kalianidis C, Markis N, Asavantinos D. Hysterosalpingography and hysteroscopy in female infertility. Hum Reprod. 1994;9:2353–5.
2. Ait Benkaddour Y, Gervaise A, Fernandez H. Which is the method of choice for evaluating uterine cavity in infertility workup? Gynecol Obstet Biol Reprod. 2010;39(8):606–13.
3. Fabres C, Alam V, Balmaceda J. Comparison of ultrasonography and hysteroscopy in the diagnosis of intrauterine lesions in infertile women. J Am Assoc Gynecol Laparosc. 1998;5:375–8.
4. Meizner I, Shokeir TA. Predictive value of TVUS performed before routine diagnostic hysteroscopy for evaluation of infertility. Fertil Steril. 2000;37:593–610.
5. Cunha-Filho JSL, Souza CAB, Salazar CC, Facin AC, Freitas FM, Passos EP. Accuracy of HSG and hysteroscopy for diagnosis of intrauterine lesions in infertile patients in an assisted fertilization programme. Gynecol Endosc. 2001;10:45–8.
6. Bettocchi S, Nappi L, Ceci O. Office hysteroscopy. Obstet Gynecol Clin North Am. 2004;31:641–54.

7. Polisseni F, Bambirra EA, Camargos AF. Detection of chronic endometritis by diagnostic hysteroscopy in asymptomatic infertile patients. Gynecol Obstet Invest. 2003;55:205–10.
8. Doldi N, Prsico P, Di Sebastiano F, et al. Pathologic findings in hysteroscopy before in vitro fertilization-embryo transfer (IVF-ET). Gynecol Endocrinol. 2005;21:235–7.
9. Pellicano M, Guida M, Zullo F, Lavitola G, Cirillo D, Nappi C. Carbon dioxide versus normal saline as a uterine distention medium for diagnostic vaginoscopic hysteroscopy in infertile patients. Fertil Steril. 2003;79:418–21.
10. Di Spiezio Sardo A, Bettocchi S, Spinelli M, Guida M, Nappi L, Angioni S, Sosa Fernandez LM, Nappi C. Review of new office-based hysteroscopic procedures 2003-2009. J Minim Invasive Gynecol. 2010;17(4):436–48.
11. Oliveira FG, Abdelmassih VG, Diamond MP, Dozortsev D, Nagy ZP, Abdelmassih R. Uterine cavity findings and hysteroscopic interventions in patients undergoing in vitro fertilization-embryo transfer who repeatedly cannot conceive. Fertil Steril. 2003;80:1371–5.
12. Demirol A, Gurgan T. Effect of treatment of intrauterine pathologies with office hysteroscopy in patients with recurrent IVF failure. Reprod Biomed Online. 2004;8:590–4.
13. Hinckley MD, Milki AA. 1000 office-based hysteroscopies prior to in vitro fertilization: feasibility and findings. JSLS. 2004;8:103–7.
14. Rama Raju GA, Shashi KG, Krishna KM, Prakash GJ, Madan K. Assessment of uterine cavity by hysteroscopy in assisted reproduction programme and its influence on pregnancy outcome. Arch Gynecol Obstet. 2006;274:160–4.
15. Karayalcin R, Ozcan S, Moraloglu O, Ozyer S, Mollamahmutoglu L, Batioglu S. Results of 2500 office-based diagnostic hysteroscopies before IVF. Reprod BioMedicine Online. 2010;20:689–93.
16. Day Baird D, Dunson DB, Hill MC, Cousins D, Schectman JM. High cumulative incidence of uterine leiomyoma in black and white women: ultrasound evidence. Am J Obstet Gynecol. 2003;188:100–7.
17. Donnez J, Jadoul P. What are the implications of myomas on fertility? A need for a debate? Hum Reprod. 2002;17:1424–30.
18. Pritts EA. Fibroids and infertility: a systematic review of the evidence. Obstet Gynecol Surv. 2001;56:483–91.
19. Sudik R, Husch K, Steller J, Daume E. Fertility and pregnancy outcome after myomectomy in sterility patients. Eur J Obstet Gynecol Reprod Biol. 1996;65:209–14.
20. Matsuzaki S, Canis M, Darcha C, Pouly JL, Mage G. HOXA-10 expression in the mid-secretory endometrium of infertile patients with either endometriosis, uterine fibromas or unexplained infertility. Hum Reprod. 2009;24:3180–7.
21. Rackow BW, Taylor HS. Submucosal uterine leiomyomas have a global effect on molecular determinants of endometrial receptivity. Fertil Steril. 2010;93:2027–34.
22. Bosteels J, Kasius J, Weyers S, Broekmans FJ, Mol BWJ, D'Hooghe TM. Hysteroscopy for treating subfertility associated with suspected major uterine cavity abnormalities. Cochrane Database Syst Rev. 2015;2:CD009461.
23. Ben-Nagi J, Miell J, Yazbek J, Holland T, Jurkovic D. The effect of hysteroscopic polypectomy on the concentrations of endometrial implantation factors in uterine flushings. Reprod Biomed Online. 2009;19:737–44.
24. Peng X, Li T, Xia E, Xia C, Liu Y, Yu D. A comparison of oestrogen receptor and progesterone receptor expression in endometrial polyps and endometrium of premenopausal women. J Obstet Gynaecol. 2009;29:340–6.
25. Kim MR, Kim YA, Jo MY, Hwang KJ, Ryu HS. High frequency of endometrial polyps in endometriosis. J Am Assoc Gynecol Laparosc. 2003;10:46–8.
26. de Sa Rosa e de Silva AC, Rosa e Silva JC, Candido dos Reis FJ, Nogueira AA, Ferriani RA. Routine office hysteroscopy in the investigation of infertile couples before assisted reproduction. J Reprod Med. 2005;50:501–6.
27. Perez-Medina T, Bajo-Arenas J, Salazar F, Redondo T, Sanfrutos L, Alvarez P, Engels V. Endometrial polyps and their implication in the pregnancy rates of patients undergoing intrauterine insemination: a prospective, randomized study. Hum Reprod. 2005;20:1632–5.

28. Varasteh NN, Neuwirth RS, Levin B, Keltz MD. Pregnancy rates after hysteroscopic polypectomy and myomectomy in infertile women. Obstet Gynecol. 1999;94:168–71.
29. Spiewankiewicz B, Stelmachow J, Sawicki W, Cendrowski K, Wypych P, Swiderska K. The effectiveness of hysteroscopic polypectomy in cases of female infertility. Clin Exp Obstet Gynecol. 2003;30:23–5.
30. Shokeir TA, Shalan HM, El-Shafei MM. Significance of endometrial polyps detected hysteroscopically in eumenorrheic infertile women. J Obstet Gynaecol Res. 2004;30:84–9.
31. Devi Wold AS, Pham N, Arici A. Anatomic factors in recurrent pregnancy loss. Semin Reprod Med. 2006;24:25–32.
32. Romero R, Espinoza J, Mazor M. Can endometrial infection/inflammation explain implantation failure, spontaneous abortion, and preterm birth after in vitro fertilization? Fertil Steril. 2004;82:799–804.
33. Feghali J, Bakar J, Mayenga JM, Segard L, Hamou J, Driguez P, Belaisch-Allart J. Systematic hysteroscopy prior to in vitro fertilization. Gynecol Obstet Fertil. 2003;31:127–31.
34. Varma TR. Genital tuberculosis and subsequent fertility. Int J Gynaecol Obstet. 1991;35:1–11.
35. Kodaman PH, Arici A. Intrauterine adhesions and fertility outcome: how to optimize success? Curr Opin Obstet Gynecol. 2007;19(3):207–14.
36. Garbin O, Ziane A, Castaigne V, Rongières C. Do hysteroscopic metroplasties really improve reproductive outcome? Gynecol Obstet Fertil. 2006;34(9):813–8.
37. Mollo A, De Franciscis P, Colacurci N, Cobellis L, Perino A, Venezia R, Alviggi C, De Placido G. Hysteroscopic resection of the septum improves the pregnancy rate of women with unexplained infertility: a prospective controlled trial. Fertil Steril. 2009;91(6):2628–31.
38. Taylor E, Gomel V. The uterus and fertility. Fertil Steril. 2008;89(1):1–16.
39. Bosteels J, Weyers S, Puttemans P, Panayotidis C, Van Herendael B, Gomel V, Mol BW, Mathieu C, D'Hooghe T. The effectiveness of hysteroscopy in improving pregnancy rates in subfertile women without other gynaecological symptoms: a systematic review. Hum Reprod Update. 2010;16:1–11.
40. El-Toukhy T, Sunkara SK, Coomarasamy A, Grace J, Khalaf Y. Outpatient hysteroscopy and subsequent IVF cycle outcome: a systematic review and meta-analysis. Reprod Biomed Online. 2008;16:712–9.
41. Nastri CO, Lensen SF, Gibreel A, Raine-Fenning N, Ferriani RA, Bhattacharya S, et al. Endometrial injury in women undergoing assisted reproductive techniques. Cochrane Database Syst Rev. 2015;3:CD009517.
42. Pundir J, Pundir V, Omanwa K, Khalaf Y, El-Toukhy T. Hysteroscopy prior to the first IVF cycle: a systematic review and meta-analysis. Reprod Biomed Online. 2014;28:151–61.
43. Dhulkotia J, Coughlan C, Li TC, Ola B. Effect of endometrial injury on subsequent pregnancy rates in women undergoing IVF after previous implantation failure: systematic review and meta-analysis. BJOG. 2012;119:132–3.
44. El-Toukhy T, Sunkara S, Khalaf Y. Local endometrial injury and IVF outcome: a systematic review and meta-analysis. Reprod Biomed Online. 2012;25:345–54.
45. Potdar N, Gelbaya T, Nardo LG. Endometrial injury to overcome recurrent embryo implantation failure: a systematic review and meta-analysis. Reprod Biomed Online. 2012;25:561–71.
46. Li R, Hao G. Local injury to the endometrium: its effect on implantation. Cur Opin. Obstet Gynecol. 2009;21:236–9.
47. Haider S, Knöfler M. Human tumor necrosis factor: physiological and pathological roles in placenta and endometrium. Placenta. 2009;30:111–23.
48. Gnainsky Y, Granot I, Aldo PB, Barash A, Or Y, Schechtman E, et al. Local injury of the endometrium induces an inflammatory response that promotes successful implantation. Fertil Steril. 2010;94:2030–6.
49. Díaz-Gimeno P, Horcajadas JA, Martínez-Conejero JA, Esteban FJ, Alama P, Pellicer A, et al. A genomic diagnostic tool for human endometrial receptivity based on the transcriptomic signature. Fertil Steril. 2011;95:50–60.

50. Díaz-Gimeno P, Ruiz-Alonso M, Blesa D, Bosch N, Martínez-Conejero JA, Alama P, et al. The accuracy and reproducibility of the endometrial receptivity array is superior to histological dating as diagnostic method for the endometrial factor. Fertil Steril. 2013;99:508–17.
51. Kilani Z. Live birth after hysteroscopic-guided embryo transfer: a case report. Fertil Steril. 2009;91:2733.e1–2.
52. Abou-Setta AM, Al-Inany HG, Mansour RT, Serour GI, Aboulghar MA. Effectiveness of hysteroscopic embryo transfer: a systematic review and meta-analysis with an indirect comparison of randomized trials. Fertil Steril. 2005;84:S363.
53. Strandell A, Lindhard A, Waldenström U, Thorburn J, Janson PO, Hamberger L. Hydrosalpinx and IVF outcome: a prospective, randomized multicentre trial in Scandinavia on salpingectomy prior to IVF. Hum Reprod. 1999;14(11):2762–9.
54. Darwish AM, El Saman AM. Is there a role for hysteroscopic tubal occlusion of functionless hydrosalpinges prior to IVF/ICSI in modern practice. Acta Obstet Gynecol Scand. 2007;86(12):1484–9.
55. Visser DS, Fourie F, Kruger HF. Multiple attempts at embryo transfer: effect on pregnancy outcome in an *in vitro* fertilization and embryo transfer program. J Assist Reprod Genet. 1993;10:37–43.
56. Noyes N. Hysteroscopic cervical canal shaving: a new therapy for cervical stenosis before embryo transfer in patients undergoing *in vitro* fertilization. Fertil Steril. 1999;71:965–6.
57. Mahajan N, Gupta I. Use of Versapoint to refashion the cervical canal to overcome unusually difficult embryo transfers and improve in-vitro fertilization-embryo transfer outcome: a case series. J Hum Reprod Sci. 2011;4(1):12–6.

Hysteroscopy in Tubal Disease

10

Dattaprasad B. Inamdar

10.1 Introduction

Tubal disease is an important cause of infertility, responsible for 25–35% cases of female causes of infertility [1]. The fallopian tube plays an important role in the mechanical transport and physiological sustenance of the gametes and early conceptus. Both normal anatomy (patent tubes, no peritubal adhesion) and physiological function (coordinated neuromuscular activity, ciliary action, and endocrine secretions) are required for successful tubal function. Consequently tubal factor infertility can be due to anatomical disturbances (stenoocclusion) or altered physiological function (changes in the tubal mucosal lining or muscular wall).

The tubal disease causing infertility can be classified as proximal, midtubal, distal, or combination of the three depending on location of tubal damage.

Of all the tubal diseases, those amenable to some treatment by hysteroscopy are proximal tubal occlusion caused either by debris, mucous plugs, or blood clots and of course sometimes to rule out tubal spasm giving false impression of tubal block and the distal tubal disease in the form of hydrosalpinx with blocked fimbrial end.

Midtubal disease is generally due to intense fibrosis due to PID/surgical intervention or congenital and is not amenable to treatment by hysteroscopy.

10.2 Hysteroscopy in Proximal Tubal Disease

Hysterosalpingography (HSG) is considered as first-line investigation for evaluation of tubal patency and to rule out tubal obstruction.

Though negative predictive value of HSG is >97%, it has low positive predictive value in tubal obstruction of 50–85% [2].

D. B. Inamdar, MS, DNB, FNB (Rep Med)
Department of Obstetrics and Gynecology, Bharati Vidyapeeth (Deemed to be University)
Medical College, Pune, Maharashtra, India

© Springer Nature Singapore Pte Ltd. 2018
S. Jain, D. B. Inamdar (eds.), *Manual of Fertility Enhancing Hysteroscopy*,
https://doi.org/10.1007/978-981-10-8028-9_10

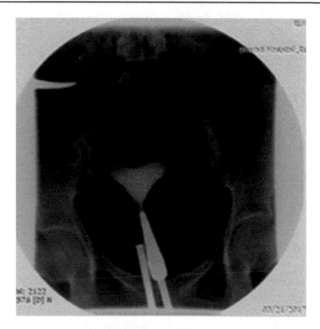

Fig. 10.1 HSG showing B/L cornual block (Courtesy: Department of Radiology, Bharati Hospital, BVUMC, Pune)

This especially happens due to false/pseudo-blocks due to cornual spasm and can happen with mucous plugs, debris, clots, salpingitis isthmica nodosa, or due to true obstruction caused by fibrosis secondary to PID or genital tuberculosis.

Hysteroscopy comes to our rescue when HSG shows cornual block. Unless it's true block due to fibrosis or due to SIN, it should be amenable to hysteroscopic tubal cannulation and attempt to open up the tube.

10.2.1 Indication of Hysteroscopic Tubal Cannulation

When HSG/hystero-salpingo contrast sonography (HyCoSy) shows unilateral or bilateral cornual block (Fig. 10.1) and there is no other indication of IVF or patient is unwilling for IVF, an attempt to open the tube through hysteroscopic tubal cannulation can be made.

Generally hysteroscopic tubal cannulation or cornual catheterization is done along with laparoscopy to know success or failure by direct visualization of free spill or its absence.

10.2.2 Contraindications

1. Active pelvic infection including active pelvic TB.
2. If there are other indications for in vitro fertilization/intracytoplasmic sperm injection (IVF/ICSI) like oligoasthenoteratozoospermia (OATS), reduced

ovarian reserve, patient undergoing preimplantation genetic diagnosis/screening (PGD/PGS) for genetic indications and patient is willing for same, cannulation shouldn't be attempted.

3. When tubes appear unhealthy or there is tubo-ovarian mass seen on laparoscopy, cannulation is futile.

4. When laparoscopy confirms strictures at multiple sites.

10.2.3 Procedure

10.2.3.1   Instrumentation

(a) Any hysteroscope with operative channel and preferably 30° angle of vision can be used.

(b) Catheter for tubal cannulation. Any tubular catheter of sufficient flexibility and diameter can be used for cannulation. Wide variety catheter/cannulation systems have been in use, including ureteric catheter, angioplasty catheter, epidural catheter, infant feeding tube, embryo transfer catheter, specialized coaxial catheters like Novy (Cook), Terumo guide wires, etc.

The choice of particular cannulation depends on individual preference, cost, and availability. Although coaxial systems are safer and easier to operate, these are costly and not widely available. Simplest and cost-effective cannulation system is that of ureteric catheters (Fig. 10.2) with or without guide wire. It's cheap and easily available, though risk of tubal perforation might be slightly higher theoretically than coaxial systems.

(c) Irrigation system with normal saline, hysteromat, laparoscopy set with telescope, light system, camera, etc.

10.2.3.2   Technique

Laparoscopy can be performed first to know whether tubal block really exists, as 25–50% blocks are false ones occurring due to tubal spasms and do not require any intervention. It also rules out contraindications for the procedure like unhealthy tubes, multiple tubal strictures, hydrosalpinx, etc. Additionally it also helps in checking success or failure of the intervention.

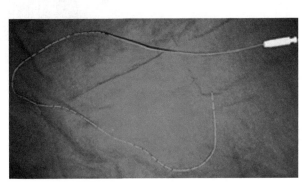

Fig. 10.2 Ureteric catheter of 3.5–5 Fr can be used for cannulation

Dilute methylene blue/indigo carmine dye should be used to test tubal patency before attempting tubal cannulation to avoid dark staining of endometrium and obscured view of subsequent hysteroscopy.

Once cornual block is confirmed and nature and health of tubes are known, decision to proceed with cornual catheterization is made.

One should be conversant with hysteroscopy and tubal anatomy before attempting tubal cannulation. Normally tubal ostia are seen as membranous rings with sharp edge on either side in cornual region. If there is any obvious pathology blocking ostium and obstructing flow of dye (like small polyp or membranous adhesions), same should be removed, and tubal patency tested once more before attempting tubal cannulation, as cannulation may no longer be needed in case of patent tubes.

Once it is confirmed to be cornual obstruction, one can proceed with cannulation.

Using 30° hysteroscope, one ostium is brought in focus in such a way that ostium remains at the center of focused image. The preferred catheter (author prefers ureteric catheter either with or without guide wire, being cheap and easily available) should be introduced through operative channel of hysteroscope. The catheter is slowly pushed through ostium for 0.5–2 cm beyond ostium or until resistance to its passage is encountered (Fig. 10.3). Once the position of catheter is confirmed to be in interstitial portion of tube, dye can be pushed and spill or otherwise can be confirmed through laparoscopy. Mild blocks due to the presence of mucous plugs/debris/clot should be cleared by pressure of dye alone. If not, guide wire can be passed through catheter to dislodge the material and establish tubal patency. The most common mistake that happens is the use of excessive force leading to tubal perforation.

The procedure in case of coaxial catheters is slightly different but is similar to the one used in other coaxial systems in medical field. The coaxial system consists of guide wire, inner catheter, and outer catheter. First, the guide wire is loaded into

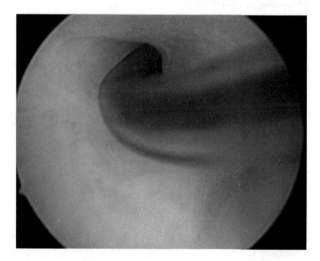

Fig. 10.3 Hysteroscopic cannulation of ostium (Courtesy: Dr. Parag Hitnalikar)

inner cannula which in turn is loaded into outer cannula. The whole cannulation set is loaded into the operative channel of hysteroscope. Once the ostium is brought into center of vision, outer catheter is advanced, which fits the uterotubal angle at the ostium. Guide wire and inner catheter are advanced into the ostium for 2–3 cm. Once the position is confirmed in the interstitial portion of the tube, guide wire is removed holding inner and outer catheters to avoid accidental withdrawal and tubal patency checked by flushing dye through inner catheter. Though the system is ideal for tubal cannulation, the set is expensive and delicate preventing widespread adoption of the system.

10.2.3.3 Complications

Apart from anesthetic complications and nonspecific complications that can occur in any hysteroscopic procedure like bleeding, infection, injury to surrounding organs, etc., the complication that is specific to tubal cannulation procedure is tubal perforation. The incidence of tubal perforation depends on ease of procedure, nature of block, and most importantly operator's skill. The incidence varies between 0% and 7% [3]. The most common cause of perforation is the use of excessive force to negotiate resistance, the other being wrong direction of catheter. It can be avoided by not using of force when resistance is encountered, as resistance in most cases indicates irreversible obstruction due to fibrosis. Most of the times, perforation heals spontaneously and doesn't need any specific treatment. In case of excessive bleeding, hemostasis can be achieved by applying pressure with bowel grasper via laparoscopy. Risk of tubal pregnancy after procedure depends on overall tubal health and is thought to vary between 0% and 10% [5, 7].

10.2.4 Outcomes

1. Chance of success as measured by tubal patency: It varies with the cause of obstruction which can be different in the different subsets of patients and varies between 37% and 80% [3–6].
2. Chance of pregnancy in case of successful patency: Varies between 20% and 73% and depends on multiple factors other than tubal patency [3, 5, 7, 8].
3. The overall mean time to become pregnant from natural conception or via clomiphene induction after successful unilateral or bilateral hysteroscopic cannulation varies between 10.5 [6] and 16.2 months [8].
4. Durability of effect: Chances of reocclusion in 1 year is 25% overall (67% in nonpregnant women) [7]. Most of the pregnancies after tubal cannulation happen within first 6 months after successful cannulation, though pregnancy can occur as late as 24 months after cannulation.
5. Chance of ectopic pregnancy: Depends on overall health of tubes and is quoted to vary between 0% and 10% [5, 7].
6. How does it compare against IVF: There has not been any study comparing hysteroscopic tubal cannulation with IVF as far as cost is concerned.

10.3   Hysteroscopy in Distal Tubal Disease

10.3.1 Hysteroscopy for Hydrosalpinx

The presence of hydrosalpinx (Fig. 10.4) adversely affects fertility both naturally and after IVF. How hydrosalpinx reduces fertility is unknown. The hydrosalpinx fluid is thought to be embryotoxic due to lack of nutrients and high reactive oxygen species (ROS) levels, or it can alter endometrial receptivity or have mechanical effect. Initial studies of salpingectomy prior to IVF and to increase fertility naturally by removing one hydrosalpingotic tube gave encouraging results. As salpingectomy can reduce ovarian blood supply and hence ovarian reserve, less radical surgeries of delinking tube from uterine end (tubal clipping) were attempted which gave equally good results and devoid of effect on ovarian blood supply.

Going by same philosophy, blocking cornual end of tube can be attempted to mimic effect of tubal clipping without need of laparoscopy. The occlusion of ostia through hysteroscopy can be achieved by using monopolar/bipolar current [9], microemboli, silicon plugs, or more recently Essure device.

Hysteroscopic occlusion of ostia can be performed in an infertile woman when:

1. Laparoscopy is contraindicated due to anaesthesia/surgical risk.
2. There are dense adhesions around tubes, making it inaccessible through laparoscopy for clipping/salpingectomy.
3. Refusal for laparoscopy by the patient.

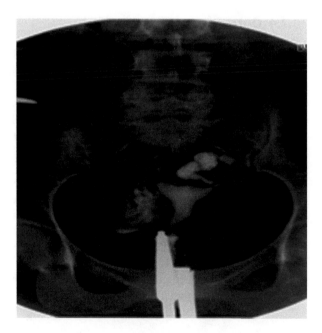

Fig. 10.4 HSG—
Hydrosalpinx (Courtesy:
Department of Radiology,
Bharati Hospital, BVUMC,
Pune)

Hong-Chu Bao et al. [9] used monopolar current of 40–60 W for 5–10 s with roller ball of 3 mm to cauterize and block the ostium on the side affected by hydrosalpinx. Though no complication was reported in the ten patients who underwent the procedure, it should not be attempted by novice surgeons for the fear of cornual perforation and thermal damage to the tubes, uterus, and sometimes beyond it (to bowel/bladder).

10.3.2   Placement of Essure Hysteroscopically

Essure (Fig. 10.5) was introduced as a method of sterilization and was approved by FDA way back in 2002. It prevents pregnancy by blocking cornual end of the fallopian tube. Though its use was theoretically possible in treating hydrosalpinx before IVF, there were (and are) concerns that the coils projecting in uterine cavity can hinder implantation or lead to miscarriage [10]. In 2005, Rosenfield et al. [11] reported first successful pregnancy and subsequently live birth in an obese woman (body mass index >50 kg/m^2) with a hydrosalpinx and extensive pelvic adhesions following use of Essure before IVF. Since then there have been multiple case reports and case series on the use of Essure to treat hydrosalpinx before IVF.

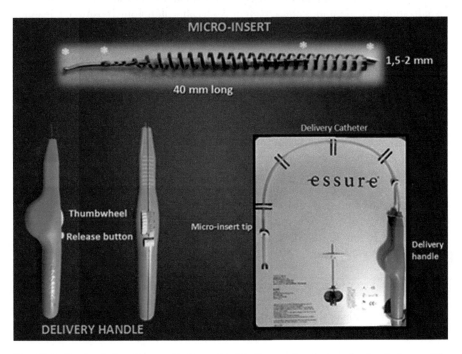

Fig. 10.5 Essure device (Source: Radiographic Findings and patient evaluation in irreversible fallopian tube occlusion contraceptive device Essure; EPOS™; ECR 2014/C-0576; reproduced with permission from Javier Azpeitia Armán) [16]

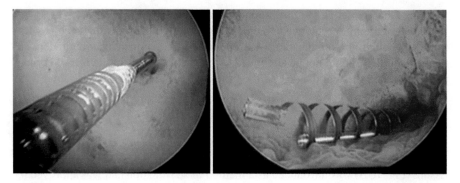

Fig. 10.6 Essure device before placement (left) and after placement with five coils trailing in cavity (right) (Source: Radiographic Findings and patient evaluation in irreversible fallopian tube occlusion contraceptive device Essure; EPOS™; ECR 2014/C-0576; reproduced with permission from Javier Azpeitia Armán) [16]

10.3.3 Procedure of Essure Placement

Essure placement (Fig. 10.6) can be done as outpatient procedure. After written informed consent and ruling out contraindications (active pelvic infection, pregnancy, allergy to nickel, patients who have known abnormal uterine cavity making visualization of ostia impossible), patient is placed in lithotomy position. Cleaning with antiseptic solution and draping follow abdominal and bimanual vaginal examination to confirm position of uterus making dilatation of cervix easy if required.

Either cervix can be held with the help of speculum and Allis/vulsellum or vaginoscopic approach can be used to introduce hysteroscope of a diameter of 4–5.5 mm with 15/30° angle. Whole uterine cavity and both ostia are visualized for feasibility of procedure. Scope is rotated at 45°, and one of the ostium is brought to the center of visual field.

Once an ostium is brought to the center of visual field, the Essure catheter is advanced through operating channel into the ostium till black positioning marker is seen at the ostium. Thumbwheel of handle is rotated and rolled back until it reaches hard stop, and the gold band can be seen. Once done, pressing the button on the thumbwheel and rolling it back detach the insert allowing it to expand in the fallopian tube. Three to eight coils trailing into the uterine cavity indicates successful placement of Essure device (Fig. 10.6). Procedure can be repeated on other side if indicated. HSG performed after 3 months verifies placement and confirms blockage.

Procedure needs to be terminated if:

1. One or both ostia or the one on the side of hydrosalpinx is not visible.
2. Excessive resistance during placement occurs (higher risk of placing it in false passage and risk of perforation).
3. Insert placement is not successful after 10 min of attempted cannulation per tube.

10.3.4 Complications of Essure Placement

Tubal/uterine perforation, failure of tubal occlusion (common in immunosuppressed patients), and allergic reaction to the material used in Essure are the possible complications apart from complications of anaesthesia, fluid overload, and discomfort/ pain due to the presence of device. Minor perforations due to sound/dilator, etc. are of no consequence if there is no excessive bleeding. If the device migrates in abdominal cavity, laparoscopy/laparotomy is required for its removal. Management of other complications is discussed elsewhere in the book.

10.3.5 Evidence and Recommendations for Clinical Practice

Studies evaluating use of Essure to treat unilateral hydrosalpinx to improve fertility are not yet available. There have been multiple case reports and case series on use of Essure to treat hydrosalpinx before IVF. These have been nicely summarized in a systemic review by P Arora et al. [12], which concludes that Essure is an effective option for management of hydrosalpinx, although evidence from randomized trials is lacking. Systematic review by Barbosa [13] had some different conclusion regarding higher miscarriage rates after Essure placement for hydrosalpinx before embryo transfer.

Without going into details of case series and meta-analyses (sadly evidence from RCTs is not available as of now to form definite guidelines), following conclusions can be drawn:

1. In case of unilateral or bilateral hydrosalpinx, laparoscopic tubal clipping/salpingectomy should be the first choice to improve fecundity either naturally or through IVF.
2. When laparoscopy is contraindicated or laparoscopic treatment is not possible due to dense adhesions or if patient refuses laparoscopy, option of Essure placement hysteroscopically should be offered.
3. When discussing option of Essure placement through hysteroscopy, possibility of higher miscarriage rate when compared to laparoscopic treatment should be discussed with the couple along with other pros and cons of Essure placement.

10.3.6 Other Methods to Treat Hydrosalpinx Through Hysteroscopy

Apart from Essure, the other method of hysteroscopic sterilization that can be used in the treatment of hydrosalpinx is Adiana. It uses bipolar radiofrequency energy within the fallopian tubes, followed by insertion of a nonabsorbable biocompatible silicone elastomer polymer matrix to promote scarring. But as there is just a single report of its use in the treatment of hydrosalpinx, it's not elaborated in detail in the present chapter.

10.4 Hysteroscopy for Tubal Evaluation: Falloscopy

Falloscopy is visualization of the fallopian tubes via a microendoscope. It can be done through hysteroscopy in case of coaxial systems and without the need of hysteroscopy/laparoscopy in case of linear everting systems. The main purpose of falloscopy in infertile women was to diagnose and treat subtle tubal abnormalities like flimsy adhesions and removal of debris/clots, to diagnose pseudo-obstructions due to spasms and to see health of tubal endothelium for prognostication. But with the advent of IVF/ICSI and increasing success rates achieved with ART procedures, the need for such invasive procedure has gone in dispute, especially considering the fact that full evaluation of tubes was possible only in <57% of cases in a large prospective international multicenter study by Rimbach et al. [14] and the plan of management (either intrauterine insemination in stimulated cycle or IVF) rarely depends exclusively on its findings.

10.5 Novel Use of Hysteroscopy in Assisting Laparoscopic Tubal Recanalization (Sterilization Reversal)

Tubal sterilization procedures are the most favored methods of permanent contraception worldwide [15]. The need for sterilization reversal can arise in case of regret about decision, child loss/disability, or second marriage. Historically open microsurgical recanalization was the favored procedure. With advances in laparoscopy, increasing skills of laparoscopic surgery, and availability of laparoscopic microsurgical instruments, laparoscopic reversal of sterilization is gaining popularity.

Though detailed discussion about indications, contraindications, and benefits of laparoscopic tubal sterilization reversal procedures is out of purview of this chapter, shortly it can be summarized as follows.

Indications: Desire to conceive in a woman having undergone tubal sterilization procedure. There should be no contraindication to the procedure.

Contraindications: All those conditions where IVF will be probably giving more chance of success—e.g., associated male factor infertility, salpingectomy/fimbriectomy performed during sterilization procedure, poor ovarian reserve, unhealthy tubes, final estimated length of tubes <3–4 cm, extensive pelvic adhesions, and contraindications to surgery/pregnancy.

Advantages of laparoscopic tubal recanalization: Cosmetically better, less postoperative adhesions compared to open surgery (due to tissue handling, injury by retractors, mops, etc.), all principles of microsurgery like magnification, tissue handling, and lavage can be followed, better for training of residents as live surgery can be seen on monitor.

Though laparoscopic tubal sterilization reversal has advantages, it is technically challenging as it requires knowledge and skill of endosuturing over mobile and delicate fallopian tubes. Endosuturing without causing excess trauma to tube still remains a bottleneck in the procedure. To make the job of endosuturing simpler, we have proposed innovative use of hysteroscopic tubal cannulation systems (catheter inserted through ostium and brought out through fimbrial end through recanaliza-tion site). It ensures stability of tubes and at the same time rules out and sometimes even treats multiple site block. It can also avoid rotational misalignment at recanalization site. Author has himself tried the procedure. Though it increases time by additional hysteroscopy and cannulation, it increases ease of endosuturing and reduces time required for endosuturing. RCTs are recommended to know usefulness of the procedure in reducing operative time, increasing ease of surgery, and to know the effect on pregnancy rates after the procedure.

Conclusion

1. Proximal tubal obstructions are most likely to be false ones or due to debris/mucous plugs/clots, these can be successfully treated by hysteroscopic tubal cannulation to achieve patency.
2. Women with significant hydrosalpinx who are not desirous/fit for laparoscopic treatment can be offered hysteroscopic placement of Essure device to increase fertility.
3. Hysteroscopic assistance by tubal cannulation during laparoscopic tubal sterilizatio n reversal operations can ease endosuturing and needs further evaluation in RCTs.

References

1. Honoré GM, AEC H, Schenken RS. Pathophysiology and management of proximal tubal blockage. Fertil Steril. 1999;71(5):785–95.
2. Das S, Nardo LG, Seif MW. Proximal tubal disease: the place for tubal cannulation. Reprod Biomed Online. 2007;15:383–8.
3. Mohapatra P, Swain S, Pati T. Hysteroscopic tubal cannulation: our experience. J Obstet Gynecol Ind. 2004;54(5):498–9.
4. Mekaru K, Yagi C, Asato K, et al. Hysteroscopic tubal catheterization under laparoscopy for proximal tubal obstruction. Arch Gynecol Obstet. 2011;284:1573.
5. Maikis R, Anderson TL, Daniell JF. Hysteroscopic tubal cannulation: long-term results. Gynaecol Endosc. 2000;9(6):397–400.
6. Chung JP, Haines CJ, Kong GW. Long term reproductive outcome after hysteroscopic proximal tubal cannulation an outcome analysis. Aust N Z J Obstet Gynaecol. 2012;52(5):470–5.
7. Kamalini D, Nagel Theodore C, Malo John W. Hysteroscopic cannulation for proximal tubal obstruction: a change for the better? Fertil Steril. 1995;63(5):1009–15.
8. Al-Jaroudi D, Herba MJ, Tulandi T. Reproductive performance after selective tubal catheterization. J Minim Invasive Gynecol. 2005;12(2):150–2.
9. Bao H-C, Wang M-M, Wang X-R, Wang W-J, Hao C-F. Clinical application of operative hysteroscopy in treatment of complex hydrosalpinx prior to IVF. Iran J Reprod Med. 2015;13(5):311–6.
10. Practice Committee of ASRM. Role of tubal surgery in the era of assisted reproductive technology: a committee opinion. Fertil Steril. 2015;103(6):e37–43.
11. Rosenfield RB, Stones RE, Coates A, Matteri RK, Hesla JS. Proximal occlusion of hydrosalpinx by hysteroscopic placement of microinsert before in vitro fertilization-embryo transfer. Fertil Steril. 2005;83:1547–50.
12. Arora P, Arora RS, Cahill D. Essure for management of hydrosalpinx prior to in vitro fertilization—a systematic review and pooled analysis. BJOG. 2014;121:527–36.

13. Barbosa MW, Sotiriadis A, Papatheodorou SI, Mijatovic V, Nastri CO, Martins WP. High miscarriage rate in women treated with Essure for hydrosalpinx before embryo transfer: a systematic review and meta-analysis. Ultrasound Obstet Gynecol. 2016;48(5):556–65.
14. Stefan R, Gunther B, Diethelm W. Technical results of falloposcopy for infertility diagnosis in a large multicentre study. Hum Reprod. 2001;16(5):925–30.
15. http://www.un.org/en/development/desa/population/publications/pdf/family/worldContraceptivePatternsWallChart2013.pdf. Accessed on 16 Jun 2017.
16. Arman JA, Ramos RML, Rodríguez-Miñón PA, Arquero FS, Gómez JMG, Barez MG, Madrid/ES Radiographic findings and patient evaluation in irreversible fallopian tube occlusion contraceptive device Essure, EPOS™, ECR 2014/C-0576.

Hysteroscopy in Endometrial Tuberculosis

11

Shikha Jain

Abbreviations

AFB	Acid fast bacilli
ATT	Anti-tubercular therapy
ART	Assisted reproductive techniques
FGTB	Female genital tuberculosis
GTB	Genital tuberculosis
HSG	Hysterosalpingography
IVF	In vitro fertilization
MTB	Mycobacterium tuberculosis
NTM	Nontuberculous mycobacteria
PCR	Polymerase chain reaction
RIF	Recurrent implantation failure
SSG	Sonosalpingography
TB	Tuberculosis
USG	Ultrasonography
WHO	World Health Organization

S. Jain, MBBS, MD, FNB (Rep Med), FICOG
Dreamz IVF, New Delhi, India

© Springer Nature Singapore Pte Ltd. 2018
S. Jain, D. B. Inamdar (eds.), *Manual of Fertility Enhancing Hysteroscopy*,
https://doi.org/10.1007/978-981-10-8028-9_11

11.1   Introduction

Tuberculosis (TB) is an age old disease and continued to remain a global health problem. In 2015, there were an estimated 10.4 million new TB cases worldwide, of which 5.9 million (56%) were among men, 3.5 million (34%) among women, and 1.0 million (10%) among children. Six countries accounted for 60% of the new cases, namely, India, Indonesia, China, Nigeria, Pakistan, and South Africa. However, the number of TB deaths and the TB incidence rate continue to fall globally which needs to accelerate to a 4–5% annual decline by 2020 to reach the first milestones of the WHO's End TB Strategy which aims at ending the TB epidemic by 2030 [1].

TB is an infectious disease caused by the *Bacillus* of *Mycobacterium* genus, *most commonly M. tuberculosis*, while the other ones are *M. bovis* or *M. africanum*, etc. The primary site of TB infection is lung, but it can affect any organ of the body. The people infected with TB can present with signs and symptoms (clinical TB) or have latent or subclinical TB. Development of active disease depends on immune status of host. In most cases with good immunity, infection either clears or defensive barrier is built round the infection where bacilli lie dormant. This is called latent TB where the person is neither ill nor infectious, but whenever body's immune mechanisms are suppressed, it can manifest itself in the lungs (pulmonary TB) or spread to the other parts of the body (extrapulmonary TB). Virtually TB can involve any organ system in the body, but the most common sites of extrapulmonary tuberculosis are the lymph nodes, pleura, abdomen, bone and joints, spinal cord, brain and meninges, genitourinary tract, and miliary TB. Extrapulmonary TB accounts for 20–25% of reported cases. TB mostly affects adults in their most reproductive years; however, all age groups are at risk. Overall, a relatively small proportion (5–15%) of the estimated two to three billion people infected with *M. tuberculosis* will develop TB disease during their lifetime [1].

11.2   Female Genital TB

Genital TB was first described by Morgagni in 1744. Genital TB is virtually always secondary to active TB infection elsewhere in the body, most commonly the lungs. The latent period from primary infection to development of genital TB is quite long (5–8 years). The spread can be hematogenous (most common), lymphatic route, or directly from the contiguous intra-abdominal sites through the fallopian tubes. The incidence of TB among women attending infertility clinics is 1–2% in developed countries but much higher in developing countries like India (3–16%) [2]. Genital TB is an important cause of significant morbidity and long-term sequelae in the form of infertility in young women.

Tubercular involvement of female genital organs in order of their occurrence [3]:

- Fallopian tubes in 90–100% cases, first to be involved
- The uterus in 50–80% predominantly endometrium and occasionally the myometrium

- Ovaries in 20–30%
- The cervix in 5–15%
- The vagina and vulva in 1–2%

Women are commonly affected in their reproductive age (20–40 years). Clinical presentation of genital TB varies according to the site of involvement. The commonest presentation is infertility due to tubal blockage, whereas chronic pelvic pain, alterations in the menstrual pattern, or pelvic mass can also be the presenting complaints. Ten to 15% of women may be asymptomatic [3].

11.2.1 Endometrial TB

Involvement of the uterus in genital TB is always secondary to infection of fallopian tubes, and it's a descending infection. The peritoneal surface of the uterus may look absolutely normal or exhibit tubercles in pelvic TB. Myometrial abscesses are extremely rare. The most common presentation is tubercular endometritis which is a chronic infection. In a study of 230 patients undergoing infertility workup, 3.9% were found to have TB endometritis [4].

The clinical presentation varies according to duration of endometrial infection. In early cases the damaged endometrium sheds with menstruation, but with involvement of basal layer of endometrium, the process of regeneration stops leading to atrophy, scarring, fibrosis, and synechia formation, and finally the shape of endometrial cavity gets distorted. Hence patient may present with polymenorrhea, hypomenorrhea, oligomenorrhea, and secondary amenorrhea. Puberty menorrhagia and postmenopausal bleeding are occasionally seen in endometrial TB. Pyometra, although very rare nowadays, is seen mostly in postmenopausal women with cervical stenosis when caseating material gets collected inside the endometrial cavity.

Association of endometrial TB and sterility was first reported by Steinsickin [4]. Infertility is caused primarily due to tubal blockage, but thin endometrial lining or intrauterine adhesions and altered ovarian function are also significant contributors. Alterations in markers of implantation, poorly developed pinopodes, reduced subendometrial blood flow, and non-receptive endometrium may lead to implantation failure in in vitro fertilization (IVF) cycles in patients of genital TB. Immunohistochemical staining of endometrium during implantation window revealed decreased expression of $\alpha v \beta 3$ integrin, E-cadherin, L-selectin, MECA-79, LIF, MUC-1, and other biochemical markers of implantation in infertile patients with genital TB compared to fertile controls [5]. TB also alters the immunology by activation of antiphospholipid antibodies and production of procoagulase causing vascular thrombus formation.

11.3   Diagnosis

Early diagnosis of genital TB is very important considering its long-term impact on patient's fertility. The clinical picture can be diverse and results on imaging may vary according to stage of disease; hence high index of suspicion is required especially in countries where TB is endemic.

11.3.1 Ultrasound

On 2D USG adnexal masses, hydrosalpinx, thin irregular endometrium with fluid in the cavity, may be seen. On sonosalpingography, diagnosis of intrauterine synechia can be made. Three-dimensional USG can clearly depict the extent of synechia. Color Doppler studies are helpful in determining endometrial and subendometrial blood flow.

11.3.2 Hysterosalpingography

HSG is contraindicated in a known case of genital TB due to the risk of flaring up of infection. But if during the infertility workup patient undergoes HSG, the findings in genital TB can be very nonspecific. Unilateral or bilateral tubal block, hydrosalpinx, beaded fallopian tubes, calcifications, venous or lymphatic intravasation, and filling defects in endometrial cavity with irregular contour suggestive of intrauterine synechia are the most common findings. In some cases an obliterated, tubular, or T-shaped cavity can be seen [6]. HSG has a sensitivity of 75–80% and specificity of 50–60% in detecting endometrial pathology with high rate of false positivity as mucous, air bubble, blood, or debris may mimic filling defects.

11.3.3 Diagnostic Hysteroscopy

Endoscopic visualization of uterine cavity is considered gold standard for the diagnosis of intrauterine pathologies with the sensitivity and specificity of 100%. In early cases of genital TB where endometrium is not involved or in subclinical infection, the endometrial cavity may be normal in shape and size with bilateral ostia clearly visible [7]. As the disease progresses, hysteroscopic presentation varies as follows (Figs. 11.1, 11.2, 11.3, 11.4, 11.5, and 11.6) [8]:

1. Fibrous bands at internal os may lead to difficulty in dilatation. If severe may present as cervical stenosis.

2. Endometrium can be hyperemic or pale, shaggy, or atrophic in different stages of the disease.
3. The presence of superficial localized ulcer [9], irregular whitish spots due to tubercles, or calcific foci is very common. Caseation is a late feature. Micropolyps have also been reported in TB endometritis [10].
4. Fibrosis at fundus or around ostia.
5. Tubal ostia: The endosalpingeal folds look pale with scarring. They do not exhibit normal opening and closing motion on fluid hysteroscopy. In later stages one or both ostium may be completely obliterated.
6. Cavity may be small, shrunken, irregular, tubular, or completely fibrosed.
7. **Intrauterine adhesions (Asherman's syndrome)**: Genital TB is one of the important causes of intrauterine adhesions, responsible for about 4% of cases [11]. Grossly the adhesions may be flimsy which appear similar to surrounding endometrium or dense which are white and thick in appearance. Initially adhesions present as isolated bands, but in later stages, they become diffuse and can obliterate the cavity partially or completely. Depending upon the location, these can be central, marginal, cornual, or cervico-isthmic. Based on composition adhesions are fibrous or fibromuscular and avascular or vascular. According to all these criteria, intrauterine adhesions are classified into different grades. An Indian study reported prevalence of different grades of intrauterine adhesions in genital TB as grade I in 17.8%, grade II in 28.5%, grade III in 28.5%, and grade IV in 17.5% [12], where grading was done according to European Society of Hysteroscopy classification (1989). Till date various classification systems are proposed for intrauterine adhesions; the author follows objective scoring system by American Fertility Society (1988) which has a prognostic value (Table 11.1) [13].

Hysteroscopy score	
1–4	Stage I (mild)
5–8	Stage II (moderate)
9–12	Stage III (severe)

Intrauterine synechiae are the reason behind infertility, repeated implantation failure (RIF) in IVF cycles, and adverse obstetric outcome in the form of repeated pregnancy loss, preterm labor, and morbidly adherent placenta.

Hysteroscopy helps in evaluation of endometrial cavity in the patients undergoing IVF and embryo transfer. Negative predictive value is more than 95%.

Table 11.1 American Fertility Society classification 1988 [13]

Classification	Extent		
Cavity involved	<1/3	1/3–2/3	>2/3
Score	1	2	4
Type of adhesions	Filmy	Filmy and dense	Dense
Score	1	2	4
Menstrual pattern	Normal	Hypomenorrhea	Amenorrhea
Score	0	2	4

11.3.4 Hysteroscopic Images in Endometrial TB

Fig. 11.2 Fundal fibrosis
with partially obliterated
ostium

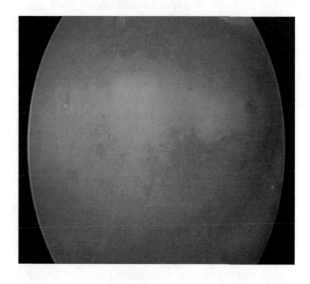

Fig. 11.1 Pale
endometrium

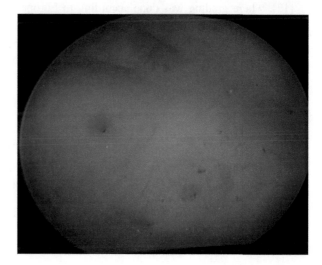

Fig. 11.3 Tubercles
(Courtesy: Dr. Parag
Hitnalikar)

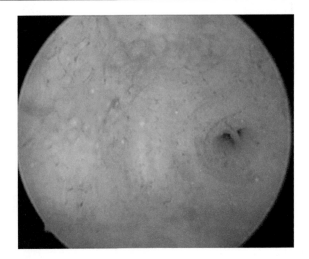

Fig. 11.4 Calcific
deposits (Courtesy Prof.
Osama Shawki and Dr.
Yehia)

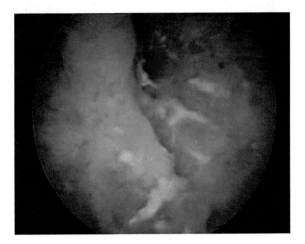

Fig. 11.5 Adhesions

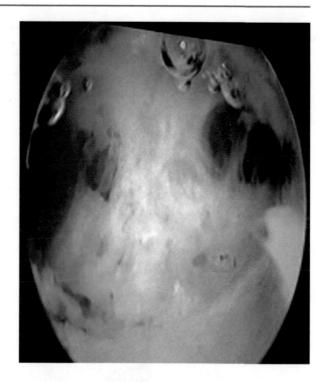

Fig. 11.6 Adhesions

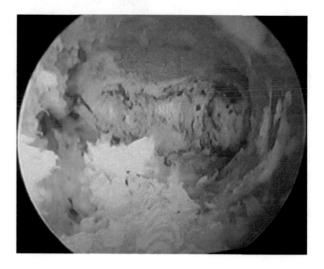

11.3.5 Histopathological

It is not possible always to have histopathological confirmation as the endometrium is involved only in 50–80% of cases of female genital TB. As the infection is descending from the fallopian tubes, cornual regions are usually the first part of the uterus to be involved. Preceding the onset of menstruation, the tubercles with bacilli are present in superficial layers of endometrium; hence premenstrual endometrial aspirate or hysteroscope directed biopsy of the endometrial tissue is sent for HPE. Demonstration of epithelioid cells, granuloma with Langerhans giant cells, is pathognomonic for TB (Fig. 11.7); however, similar picture may be seen in foreign body reaction, actinomycosis, sarcoidosis, schistosomaisis, etc. In the absence of typical granuloma or caseation, features like dilated glands, destruction of epithelium, and inflammatory lymphocytic exudate are suggestive of TB.

11.3.6 Mycobacteria-Specific Tests

Genital TB is a paucibacillary disease, so it is not possible always to demonstrate the TB bacilli. In later stages of the disease, there may be no endometrial tissue on curettage. Endometrial tissue is sent in normal saline for mycobacteria-specific tests. These tests have different sensitivity and specificity in detecting MTB, but negative test does not rule out genital TB.

1. **AFB smear**: Ziehl-Neelsen or auramine-rhodamine staining with fluorescence microscopy. 10^4–10^5 bacilli/mL are required for a positive AFB smear. The smear positivity rate is very low.
2. **AFB culture**: Tissue culture is gold standard in the diagnosis of MTB. The presence of 10–100 bacilli/mL in any sample is required for diagnosis.

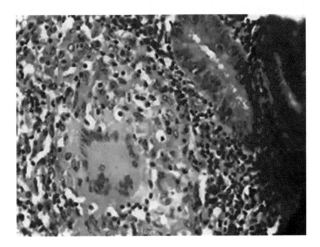

Fig. 11.7 Histopathology showing epithelioid cell granuloma with Langerhans-type giant cells in the background of inflammatory cell infiltrate (H & E section, 40×) (Courtesy Dr. Nidhi Gupta)

(a) **Lowenstein-Jensen media (solid)**: Growth is detected after 6–8 weeks. Sensitivity is lower (30–35%) [14].

(b) **AFB radiometric culture (liquid)**: Nucleic acid probes and fluorescence technology are used. The results are obtained within 10–12 days, and sensitivity is 80–90% [14].

- BACTEC 460 (Becton Dickinson & Co.): Rapid radiometric culture system
- Mycobacteria growth inhibitor tube (MGIT 960): Fluorometric, fully automated, and rapid culture system
- BacT/alert or BacT alert 3D: Colorimetric, fully automated, and rapid culture system

3. **Nucleic acid amplification tests (NAATs)**: Rapid and specific diagnosis of TB is made possible by detecting fragments of nucleic acid of *Mycobacterium tuberculosis* bacilli directly from clinical samples.

(a) **DNA PCR**: PCR targets various gene segments of mycobacterial DNA, including 65 kDa protein, IS6110 element, and MPB64 gene. It is a sensitive test which detects even 1–10 bacilli/mL, and result is obtained within 1–2 days. The sensitivity of the test is more than 90%, but the specificity is between 70% and 90%. It can detect nonviable bacilli and also positive in NTM infections and contamination. False-positive result is the biggest drawback of DNA PCR, and hence it cannot be considered as the basis to commence ATT. False negative is also very common with DNA PCR due to inadequate number of bacilli or presence of PCR inhibitors in the clinical specimen. In an endemic country like India, the PCR may be positive in healthy people as well.

   Real-time PCR is specific to IS6110 gene and remarkably decreases the incidence of false positive test.

   Gene Xpert MTB/RIF assay is a novel, cartridge-based semiautomated DNA PCR test with very high specificity which gives result within 2 h. It also detects rifampicin resistance. WHO first recommended its use in 2010, but its use in genital TB is still under evaluation [1].

(b) **mRNA PCR**: Single tube nested reverse transcription PCR directed toward 85B gene. It detects only the live organisms in the clinical specimen, but mRNA is degraded rapidly after death of bacteria (average half-life of mRNA is 3 min). Therefore the sample needs to be transported to laboratory in ice within 2 h which limits its widespread use [15]. Further its use in extrapulmonary TB is not established yet.

11.4   Treatment

Patients with active pulmonary TB, culture-proven cases of genital TB, or patients with strong clinical suspicion on laparoscopic and hysteroscopic findings should be started on anti-tubercular therapy (ATT). Author strongly recommends against starting ATT empirically, solely on the basis of positive DNA PCR or in cases of latent TB in endemic countries.

11.4.1 Medical

Genital TB is classified under category I being seriously ill extrapulmonary disease [2]. As per WHO guidelines, patients with genital TB should receive a four-drug regimen for 6 months which include:

- Intensive phase (2HRZE): Isoniazid (with pyridoxine), rifampicin, pyrazinamide, and ethambutol for 2 months
- Continuation phase (4HR): Isoniazid (with pyridoxine) and rifampicin for a further 4 months (Table 11.2)

Objective of medical management is to reduce the bacterial population followed by sterilizing the lesion. Daily dosing schedule is optimal throughout the course of therapy [16]. Three-times-weekly dosing $[2(HRZE)_3/4(HR)_3]$ is another alternative, provided that every dose is directly observed (DOTS). Fixed-dose combination tablets (FDCs) have equivalent efficacy to single pills and are more acceptable to patient. These drugs have varied side effect profile and need monitoring. Patient compliance is critically important, and incomplete or irregular treatment puts the patient at risk of relapse and development of bacterial resistance.

Medical management alone is not enough for fertility restoration in genital TB unless it is started at a very early stage of the disease, where ovarian function, tubal patency, and endometrial receptivity are not disturbed by the sequel of TB.

11.4.2 Surgical

Surgery has a limited role in the treatment of extrapulmonary TB. It is reserved for management of late sequelae of the disease such as pyometra, tubo-ovarian masses, hydrosalpinx, etc. Pelvic TB requires operative laparoscopy or laparotomy, but for endometrial TB hysteroscopic resurrection along with ATT and assisted reproductive technologies (ART) is advised.

11.4.2.1 Operative Hysteroscopy in Endometrial TB

Operative hysteroscopy is technically challenging in genital TB, owing to difficulty in finding appropriate cleavage plane, poor distension of endometrial cavity, and

Table 11.2 Recommended doses of first-line anti-tubercular drugs in adults

Drugs	Daily dose (mg/kg body weight)	Three-times-weekly dose (mg/kg body weight)
Isoniazid	5 (4–6)	10 (8–12)
Rifampicin	10 (8–12)	10 (8–12)
Pyrazinamide	25 (20–30)	35 (30–40)
Ethambutol	15 (15–20)	30 (25–35)

H, isoniazid; R, rifampicin; Z, pyrazinamide; E, ethambutol

difficulty in dilatation. Uterine perforation and accidental myometrial damage may cause uterine rupture in future pregnancy [17]. It should be scheduled in immediate postmenstrual period and preferably done under general anesthesia. While performing surgery for genital TB, fertility preservation and reconstruction should be the goal.

Dilatation of os and negotiating through cervix may release the adhesions in the cervical canal. Sometimes they are so dense which mandates division under vision. Vaginoscopic approach or office hysteroscopy with thin diameter scopes is useful in such cases. Revision of cervical canal can be performed with microscissors or electrocautery [18]. After adequate distension, the endometrial cavity and cornual regions are visualized. A note is made for the look of endometrium, whether it is pale, thinned out, or scarred. Bilateral cornua are then brought into focus to look for ostium, fibrosis, or any abnormal vasculature. Then the cavity is inspected for any suspicious lesion like ulcers, caseation, calcific foci, or tubercles. Targeted biopsy of the lesion is taken through scissors or biopsy forceps and sent for histopathological and bacteriological confirmation for the diagnosis of endometrial TB. Hemostasis is achieved through electrocautery if required. Surgeon should take extreme care while dilating the os, dividing the adhesions or excising lesions, not only to prevent perforation of the uterus but also to diagnose timely if it happens.

11.4.2.2 Synechiolysis

Tubercular intrauterine adhesions are invariably very dense and cohesive. Hysteroscopic division is considered gold standard in the management of Asherman's syndrome [19]. It can be done:

(a) Mechanically with the help of semirigid or rigid hysteroscopic scissors (5 Fr)
(b) With the help of resectoscope with monopolar (Collin's knife) or bipolar electrocautery (versapoint)
(c) Vaporization and lysis by fiberoptic lasers (Nd YAG or diode)

Flimsy adhesions are broken through hysteroscope only, but for dense fibrous adhesions, mechanical or electrosurgical instruments are used. The procedure of hysteroscopic synechiolysis is described in detail in a separate chapter, but some practical points pertaining to tubercular adhesions are described here.

Author recommends synechiolysis with hysteroscopic scissors in order to prevent damage to adjacent endometrium or devascularization which may enhance the risk of reformation of synechiae. While using resectoscope, fine electrodes should be chosen at the minimum possible current, and the adhesions are divided selectively and systematically to avoid contact with the surrounding healthy endometrium. Similar precautions apply with the use of vaporizing electrodes. When using lasers, only sculpted fibers with thin conical tips should be selected. Energy devices have the advantage of simultaneous hemostasis. It is very important to realize that the procedure should be stopped once both the ostia are visible in one plane. The aim is to restore the cavity 70–90% of normal. It can be done as a single-stage or two-stage procedure depending upon the severity of adhesions and obliteration of the cavity. Lateral metroplasty is done in small shrunken cavity. Over-resection of dense adhesions or thermal injury due to the use of electrocautery or laser can cause thinning or weakening of adjacent endometrium and/or myometrium. There is higher risk of hemorrhage and uterine perforation during synechiolysis in genital TB.

11.4.2.3 Reformation of Synechiae

Recurrence is very common in genital TB especially in women with grade III/IV adhesions [20, 21]. It ranges from 0% to 15% in mild adhesions, 16–38% in moderate, and 42–80% in severe adhesions [22]. Different measures are employed to prevent reformation of synechia like putting an intrauterine splint to keep the raw uterine walls separated. Pediatric Foley's catheter (8–10 Fr) balloon inflated with 3–5 mL saline or inert intrauterine device (e.g. Lippe's loop) has been tried. Broad spectrum antibiotics are recommended strongly whenever the splint is left in utero. Recently the use of intrauterine anti-adhesive barriers like amnion graft or auto cross-linked hyaluronic acid gel has been found effective for decreasing the recurrence of adhesions but not for increasing pregnancy or live birth rates [23]. To aid in the rapid re-epithelization of the uterine cavity, estrogen therapy in the form of estradiol valerate 4–8 mg/day or conjugated estrogen (Premarin) 0.625–5 mg daily is prescribed for 3–4 weeks. This is followed by medroxyprogesterone acetate 10 mg once a day for the last 7–10 days to induce withdrawal bleeding. Sequential estrogen—progesterone therapy should be given for minimum 3 months before proceeding for conception or second-look hysteroscopy. Second-look hysteroscopy is performed after 3–6 months of primary procedure to evaluate the contour of endometrial cavity, endometrial regeneration, and simultaneously dividing the reformed adhesions.

11.4.2.4 Results

Normal menstruation has been reestablished in over 90% of patients treated for intrauterine adhesions, but the reproductive outcome is inversely proportional to the severity of the disease. Clinical pregnancy rates range from 40% to 60%, miscarriage rates 15–20%, and live birth rates range from 25% to 50%. In general, better success rates were associated with less severe disease; the more extensive and thicker are the adhesions, the poorer is the prognosis. However, successful pregnancies have been reported even with markedly scarred uteri.

11.4.2.5 Difficulties and Complications

Though hysteroscopy is generally a simple, safe, and easy procedure, level of difficulty and complication rate might be higher in women with genital TB. Intrauterine adhesions and fibrosis, cervical stenosis and distorted cavity can cause difficulty in dilatation, formation of false passage, uterine perforation, inability to distend or visualize the cavity, excessive bleeding, flare up of TB infection, and abandoning of procedure. Late complications like placenta accreta, uterine rupture, postpartum hemorrhage, need of manual removal of placenta, or cesarean hysterectomy can occur in future pregnancy.

   In a retrospective analysis, Sharma et al. found that in patients with genital TB, there is significantly higher incidence of complications compared to those without genital TB (31.31% vs. 3.81%, $p < 0.05$). In a subgroup analysis of infertile women, similar pattern was noted (12.12% vs. 2.08%) [24].

- Inability to distend cavity in 8.08% vs. 0.69% ($p = 0.02$)
- Inability to visualize cavity in 90.9% vs. 1.04% ($p = 0.03$)
- Excessive bleeding in 5.05% vs. 0.35% ($p = 0.04$)
- Uterine perforation in 8.08% vs. 1.73% ($p = 0.008$)
- Flare up of TB 1.01% ($p = 0.04$)

Considering the risks, author recommends a thorough preoperative workup and careful selection of cases for hysteroscopic surgery in genital TB. It should be done with extreme caution, preferably by an experienced surgeon under laparoscopic guidance, in a fully equipped setup to deal with complications if any.

11.5   Fertility Outcome in Genital TB

Fertility outcome in genital tuberculosis is not optimistic. It depends upon extent and severity of the disease. In early stage disease with mild tubal damage but preserved ovarian and endometrial function, the fertility potential is comparable to general population. But with progression of disease to bilateral tubal damage and endometrial distortion, the chances of spontaneous conception are minimal. These patients are more prone to ectopic pregnancies and spontaneous abortions. Full course of ATT followed by in vitro fertilization (IVF) is the only realistic option for successful conception in these patients provided the uterine cavity, endometrial thickness, and endometrial receptivity are not compromised. Although with improvements in surgical techniques and recent advancements to improve results in IVF programs, the chances of successful conception have increased but still lower clinical pregnancy, and live birth rate per transfer is major deterrent in patients of genital TB. Various authors have reported the pregnancy rate in IVF cycles ranging from 9.1% to 38.3% and the live birth rate from 16% to 40% [25]. Gestational surrogacy or adoption should be offered in the cases with irreversible endometrial damage.

Conclusion

Genital tuberculosis is a complex disease which interferes with human conception in more than one way. The disease hampers fertility by damaging the vital reproductive organs of the female body like fallopian tubes and the uterus. Early diagnosis and timely initiation of therapeutic interventions may protect future fertility and prevent from irreparable sequel of the disease. Hysteroscopy has an important role in diagnosing the disease as well as correcting the imprints that the disease has leftover. Although the hysteroscopic restoration of endometrial cavity is not up to 100% but with advances in surgical techniques, measures to prevent recurrences coupled with the use of assisted reproductive techniques, more and more women are now being able to achieve successful conception.

References

1. World Health Organization. Global Tuberculosis Control. Global tuberculosis report 2016. 978241565394_end.pdf. Accessed on 24 Jan 2017. http://www.who.int/tb/publications/global_report/en/. World Health Organization.
2. WHO. A short update to the 2009 Report. WHO/HTM/TB/2009. 426. Geneva: WHO; 2009.
3. Sharma JB. Tuberculosis and gynecological practice. In: Studd J, Tan SL, Chervenak FA, editors. Current progress in obstetrics and gynecology, vol. 18. Mumbai: Tree Life India; 2012. p. 304–27.
4. Kajal BP, Anand AS, Trupti VK. Tuberculous endometritis - a worrying recrudescence for infertility. Int J Biol Med Res. 2012;3(2):1708–11.
5. Chakravarty BN. Female genital tuberculosis-diagnostic dilemma, management. In: Chakravarty BN, editor. Clinics in reproductive medicine and assisted reproductive technology, vol. 2. 1st ed. Delhi: CBS; 2017. p. 183–203.
6. Afzali N, Ahmadi F, Akhbari F. Various hysterosalpingography findings of female genital tuberculosis: a case series. Iran J Reprod Med. 2013;11(6):519–24.
7. Sharma JB, Roy KK, Pushparaj M, Kumar S. Hysteroscopic findings in women with primary and secondary infertility due to genital tuberculosis. Int J Gynaecol Obstet. 2009;104(1):49–52.
8. Arpitha VJ, Savitha C, Nagarathnamm R. Diagnosis of genital tuberculosis: correlation between polymerase chain reaction positivity and laparoscopic findings. Int J Reprod Contracept Obstet Gynecol. 2016;5(10):3425–32.
9. Xu D, Xue M, Han X. Hysteroscopic images of early-stage endometrial tuberculosis. Gynecol Surg. 2009;6:51–2.
10. Scrimin F, Limone A, Wiesenfeld U, Guaschino S. Tubercular endometritis visualized as endometrial micropolyps during hysteroscopic procedure. Arch Gynecol Obstet. 2010;281(6):1079–80.
11. Schenker JG, Margalioth EJ. Intrauterine adhesions: an updated appraisal. Fertil Steril. 1982;37:593–610.
12. Sharma JB, Roy KK, Pushparaj M, Gupta N, Jain SK, Malhotra N, Mittal S. Genital tuberculosis: an important cause of Asherman's syndrome in India. Arch Gynecol Obstet. 2008;277(1):37–41.
13. The American Fertility Society classifications of adnexal adhesions, distal tubal occlusion, tubal occlusion secondary to tubal ligation, tubal pregnancies, mullerian anomalies and intrauterine adhesions. Fertil Steril. 1988;49:944–55.
14. Neonakis IS, Spandidos DA, Petinaki E. Female genital tuberculosis: a review. Scand J Infect Dis. 2011;43:564–72.
15. Therese KL, Gayathri R, Dhanurekha L. R. Sridhar et al. Detection of Mycobacterium tuberculosis directly from sputum specimens & phenotypic drug resistance pattern of M. tuberculosis isolates from suspected tuberculosis patients in Chennai. Indian J Med Res. 2012;135(5):778–82.
16. NICE guideline Tuberculosis (NG 33). 2016. nice.org.uk/guidance/ng33. Accessed on 24 Jan 2017.
17. Gürgan T, Yarali H, Urman B, Dagli V, Dogan L. Uterine rupture following hysteroscopic lysis of synechiae due to tuberculosis and uterine perforation. Hum Reprod. 1996;11(2):291–3.
18. Suen Michael WH, Bougie O, Singh SS. Hysteroscopic management of a stenotic cervix. Fertil Steril. 2017;107(6):e19.
19. Magos A. Hysteroscopic treatment of Asherman's syndrome. Reprod Biomed Online. 2002;4(Suppl 3):46–51.
20. Bukulmez O, Yarali H, Gurgan T. Total corporal synechiae due to tuberculosis carry a very poor prognosis following hysteroscopic synechialysis. Hum Reprod. 1999;14(8):1960–1.
21. Bahadur A, Malhotra N, Mittal S, Singh N, Gurunath S. Second-look hysteroscopy after antitubercular treatment in infertile women with genital tuberculosis undergoing in vitro fertilization. Int J Gynaecol Obstet. 2010;108(2):128–31.

22. Yang JH, Chen CD, Chen SU, Yang YS, Chen MJ. The influence of the location and extent of intrauterine adhesions on recurrence after hysteroscopic adhesiolysis. BJOG. 2016;123(4):618–23.
23. Bosteels J, Weyers S, Mol BW, D'Hooghe T. Anti-adhesion barrier gels following operative hysteroscopy for treating female infertility: a systematic review and meta-analysis. Gynecol Surg. 2014;11:113–27.
24. Sharma JB, Roy KK, Pushparaj M, Karmakar D, Kumar S, Singh N. Increased difficulties and complications encountered during hysteroscopy in women with genital tuberculosis. J Minim Invasive Gynecol. 2011;18(5):660–5.
25. Sharma JB. In vitro fertilization and embryo transfer in female genital tuberculosis. IVF Lite. 2015;2:14–25.

Complications of Hysteroscopy

12

Shruti Gupta

12.1 Introduction

In 1981 a German surgeon Kurt Semm from the University of Kiel performed a laparoscopic appendectomy that led to his suspension from medical practice. Semm's theory was incongruous to the prevailing surgical practice and was also touted to be unethical. In current surgical practice, there are trifling handful primarily open procedures. The explanation for the trend is improved patient safety, better electrosurgical and optical transmission devices.

Hysteroscopy is one such minimally invasive procedure that has evolved over the years to a several times safer technology. Complications are fortunately few and are mostly recounted in operative procedures, pertaining to distention media and perforating trauma. The reported incidence of acute injuries is 1.65% from the University of Kiel over a period of 2 years [1]. Other studies have reported an incidence of 0.28–5.2% [2, 3].

The commonest complications reported are false passage, perforation and fluid overload [4, 5]. Women generally tolerate hysteroscopy well and major complications are relatively few. The complications can be divided broadly pertaining to anaesthesia, positioning, distention media, and the complication of surgery itself like perforation, electrosurgical burns, infection and adhesion formation (Fig. 12.1).

12.2 Position Complications

Hysteroscopy is performed in dorsal lithotomy position using candy cane or Allen stirrups. Lithotomy position increases venous return and can result in pulmonary oedema in a susceptible patient. Crush injuries of fingers may result if fingers get

S. Gupta, MD (AIIMS), DNB, FNB
Milann Kumarapark, Bengaluru, Karnataka, India

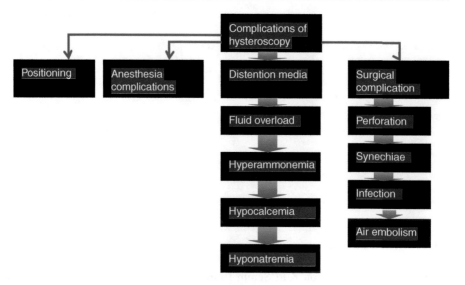

Fig. 12.1 Complications of hysteroscopy

entrapped in the break in the table. It is therefore recommended to use armrests. Neuropraxia or nerve injury is commonest to common peroneal, sciatic and saphenous nerves. The risk factors are low BMI, prolonged duration (>2 h) and cigarette use [6].

The other complication is compartment syndrome in prolonged surgeries as blood to the leg is compromised. It should be suspected in patients complaining of calf pain in the post-operative period. In prolonged surgeries padding should be used around the knees and ankles. It is also good practice to remove the legs from the stirrups if the operation is prolonged.

12.3   Anaesthesia Complications

Office and diagnostic hysteroscopy have been done with paracervical block, topical anaesthesia with or without conscious sedation. A vaginoscopic method for office hysteroscopy is also gaining popularity for reduction in pain. A combination of various methods is often used with good results in outpatient hysteroscopy [7].

Operative hysteroscopy can be performed either in general, epidural or intrathecal administered anaesthesia. The choice of the route of administration depends on the complexity and duration of the surgical procedure. Regional anaesthesia affords the advantage of the patient being awake and so can signal the early detection of fluid overload [8]. Complications due to anaesthesia are discussed in a separate chapter in this book.

12.4   Distention Media

Distention media used vary depending on the type of procedure and setup the procedure is performed in. We describe here a broad classification of distention media as described elsewhere [9].

Gaseous
  1. CO_2
Liquid media
  High molecular weight media
    1. 32% dextran 70
  Low molecular weight media
    1. Electrolyte media
        (a) Sodium chloride (NaCl)
        (b) 5% and 10% dextrose
        (c) 4% and 6% dextran
    2. Non-electrolyte media
        (a) Isotonic: 2.2% glycine, 5% mannitol, 3% sorbitol
        (b) Hypotonic: 1.5% glycine

12.4.1 Gaseous Media: CO_2

Gaseous media is best suited for diagnostic office procedures. It is a clean media for outpatient hysteroscopy. It is generally accepted that CO_2 is not appropriate for operative hysteroscopy. Endometrial debris and blood get collected and obscure the field of vision [10, 11]. Large volumes of CO_2 can get dissolved in blood with no physiologic consequences; however, when large volumes are delivered to the heart, cardiorespiratory arrest can happen as a result of CO_2 embolism. Consequently only a low-pressure hysteroscopic insufflator should only be used for cavity distention [12].

As a diagnostic distention media, CO_2 is not without demerits; according to Brusco et al., the use of anaesthesia and pain was much lower with normal saline [10].

12.4.2 Liquid Media

12.4.2.1   High Molecular Weight Media: Hyskon

This is a HMW, hyperosmolar solution of 32% dextran 70 in 10% glucose. The osmolality of the solution is high enough to cause catastrophic overload and pulmonary oedema at fluid deficit of a minimal volume ~100 mL. Dextran 70 has also an associated risk of anaphylactoid reactions, the incidence reported at 1: 821 [13].

There is caramelisation of instruments with the use of dextran and requires thorough cleaning with warm saline lest leads to spoiling of all instruments. The availability of superior distention media has limited the usage of this media.

12.4.2.2 LMW (Low Molecular Weight) Electrolyte Media

Monopolar electrosurgical devices require a non-conducting media. Usage of the monopolar device with saline disperses the current and prevents the creation of surgical effect. This leads to the usage of sterile water; however sterile water on systemic absorption can be a cause for haemolysis. The addition of solutes like glucose, sorbitol and mannitol circumvents haemolysis and provides electrolyte-free media for operative hysteroscopy.

(a) **NaCl**

Saline is ideally suited for diagnostic hysteroscopy and provides excellent image quality and better pain scores. The only problem is that spillage makes it slightly unsuitable over CO_2 for office use. Bipolar radiofrequency devices can be used with saline [14, 15]. Large volume shifts with physiological saline is well tolerated with no resulting risk of hyponatremia. However it is still imperative to maintain accurate input-output logs throughout the procedure.

(b) **Glycine**

Glycine solution is available in a concentration of 1.5% and 2.2%. This solution provides excellent clarity but has potential impact on patient safety. Glycine after absorption is metabolised in the liver into ammonia and water, which can further lead to electrolyte imbalance and water intoxication. Ammonia itself can be a cause of cerebral dysfunction as has been seen in a few cases where there was no electrolyte imbalance [16].

(c) The other solutions in use are *sorbitol*; this is an isomer of mannitol and metabolised into CO_2 and water and can cause water overload. *Mannitol* is isotonic with blood and is excreted as it is; in fact it causes an osmotic diuresis. Therefore it appears to be the safest hysteroscopic distention media in use.

12.5   Mechanism and Consequence of Intravasation, Its Prevention and Management

There are two explanations of intravasation of fluid in hysteroscopy. *Firstly* when there is vascular disruption in the myometrium and deeper endometrium, large amounts of fluid can get absorbed in the systemic circulation. *Secondly* when the distending pressure is more, the fluid moves into the vascular space. Therefore the duration that distention pressure remains over the mean arterial pressure adds to the risk of operative hysteroscopy intravasation syndrome (*OHIS*).

Menstruant women have a higher susceptibility to hyponatremia, and small values of Na^+ imbalance can lead to life-threatening cerebral oedema and cerebral herniation. The reason is that in the face of osmotic imbalance the brain compensates by removing osmotically active cations through the Na^+-K^+ ATPase pump.

This pump is inhibited in women in the reproductive age group by female sex hormones [17].

The extent and severity of OHIS can also be dependent on preexisting conditions like hypertension, heart disease and diabetes.

12.5.1 OHIS Prevention and Management

After significant absorption of fluid, the patient develops pulmonary oedema secondary to volume overload and right heart failure, which can be indicated by drop in saturation pressure, frothing and decrease in blood pressure. If the patient is in regional anaesthesia, the symptoms of vascular shift can be elucidated much earlier. The sodium deficit causes significant confusion to be noticed if the patient is in regional anaesthesia. There have been reports of laryngeal oedema necessitating tracheostomy as intubation was precluded because of the swelling [18]. The chest X-ray will show hilar infiltrates and there is a decrease in urine output. Disseminated intravascular coagulation can set in due to the hypoxia, volume overload and electrolyte imbalance [19]. Electrolyte and pH disturbances reported are primarily hyponatremia, respiratory acidosis and hyposmolality. A case of hypocalcemia and acidosis leading to ECG changes has been reported as a part of *OHIS* [20].

12.5.2 Delivery and Absorption Monitoring Systems

The simplest delivery system is a pressure fall system where the bag is hung at some elevation above the patient's uterus. Another crude modification is a pressure cuff to pump fluid, it has to be noted that though these systems provide adequate comfort for diagnostic and small procedures they offer nothing in maintaining and monitoring intrauterine pressure in other complex surgeries. The delivery systems available for this purpose overestimate the intrauterine pressure, which is also desirable as keeping intrauterine pressure below the arterial pressure decreases absorption [21, 22].

It is imperative to measure the volume deficit but is complicated by multiple factors. *Firstly* the volume in the fluid infusion bags is always more than 3 L; *secondly* the amount remaining in the bag cannot be accurately measured; *thirdly* the fluid collected on the floor and operating table cannot be measured by the theatre staff; and *finally* sometimes there may be a very rapid absorption which can compromise assessment [23].

12.5.3 Measures to Reduce Systemic Absorption

There are measures described to limit fluid absorption during the procedure, nevertheless there should be a system in place for managing fluid delivery and absorption with the help of instruments described earlier. The operating room (*OR*) staff should be able to diagnose and alert the surgeon in the event of excessive fluid absorption.

(a) *Preoperative*

GnRH analogues administered prior to procedure decrease the size and vascularity of the fibroids and endometrium. The risk of absorption is directly proportional to the size of the myoma and how deep seated in myometrium is it located. Both these factors increase the duration and the risk of vascular disruption. GnRH agonist when given can also reduce the consequence of hyponatremia as it offsets the effect of oestrogen on the $Na^+-K^+ATPase$ [24].

(b) *Intraoperative*

Vasopressin infiltration in the cervix assists in dilation of cervix and reduces vascular disruption and bleeding in the procedure. In a randomised trial including 106 women, the fluid absorption was very less when 8 mL of 0.05 U/mL of solution was infiltrated into the cervical stroma [25].

As has been discussed earlier, the selection of distention media that is safe and suitable for the procedure is an important determinant for the prevention of OHIS. The pressure of distention should be maintained below the arterial pressure, and suction devices connected to the outlet help maintain the pressure ~80–100 mmHg [26].

Resection technique using bipolar cautery or mechanical morcellation also eliminate the dangers of electrolyte imbalance [27]. During the procedure if bleeding is encountered, it usually is a warning that a major sinus is opened and precedes significant volume absorption. The procedure should be halted for 10 min, and this usually stops the bleeding and decreases fluid shift [28].

12.5.4 Management of OHIS

Apart from procedures and checks to prevent and diagnose promptly the development of volume overload, a cut-off to start resuscitation is to be established. A volume deficit of 500 mL has been reported to cause cerebral oedema. Therefore the practice of doing a CT scan in all such patients post-operatively is recommended [29]. There is no data available on the minimal fluid deficit for pulmonary oedema, but it is generally agreed that <1000 mL of electrolyte-free fluid is well tolerated by healthy premenopausal adult women. The placement of central vascular line in patients at risk of osmotic imbalance is advocated, and monitoring of electrolytes should be done after 30 mins of the procedure. A fluid deficit of 1000 mL is accompanied by decrease of 10 mmol/L of Na^+ [29]. An indwelling Foley catheter for monitoring urine output should be kept, and injection furosemide should be administered if there is intravasation of hypotonic fluids in excess of 500 mL.

Fluid overload and cardiovascular decompensation present with declining saturation and increased airway pressure. This should be managed with diuresis, ionotropes and invasive ventilation. The hyponatremia and acidosis have to be corrected with hypertonic saline and calcium carbonate.

12.6   Air Embolism

Air embolism has been reported during diagnostic as well as operative hysteroscopy [30]. The source of air embolism is room air or air in the tubing or pressurised infusion of distending media; otherwise when CO_2 is used, embolism can result. When the patient is put in Trendelenburg position, the venous pressure decreases and the air can get sucked in to the venous circulation. It is therefore advised not to perform hysteroscopy in Trendelenburg position.

When embolism occurs it is usually indicated by a drop in saturation and decrease blood pressure due to hypotention secondary to right heart failure. Other monitoring systems when the patient is under anaesthesia are end-tidal CO_2 and trans-esophageal echocardiography. 200–300 mL of air is required to cause air embolism. This can be controlled within minutes by left lateral decubitus and administration of 100% O_2. In extreme cases air may be aspirated from the heart through a needle introduced below the left costal margin. 100% O_2 and adequate ionotropic and fluid support are required to maintain and assist recovery from haemodynamic collapse [31].

12.7   Surgical Complications

12.7.1 Perforation

Cervical lacerations during dilation occur frequently and can make subsequent operative intervention difficult. The uterine perforations also occur more commonly during dilation of cervix. The reported incidence is 1–9% of hysteroscopy cases [32]. During operative hysteroscopy, perforation occurs during myoma resection and septal resection at the completion of surgery. Whenever perforation occurs with an electrosurgical instrument, exploration is recommended to diagnose bowel or bladder injuries. The uterine perforation is sutured even if not bleeding in infertile patients and women of reproductive age to prevent uterine rupture or placental adherence [33, 34].

Perforation can be prevented by careful serial dilation of cervix and usage of vaginal misoprostol prior to the procedure. A perforation is recognised by loss of resistance and collapse of the uterine walls. The site of perforation also determines the extent of damage and its management. A midline perforation is usually of no consequence but lateral perforation risk involvement of vessels leading to formation of a retroperitoneal haematoma and must be checked on laparoscopy or laparotomy. The cornua are the weakest regions and as such require precise method of approach.

Surgeries like myomectomy, synechiolysis and septal resection have a tangible risk of perforation. Performing these procedures under laparoscopic or ultrasound guidance can reduce the risk considerably [35].

12.7.2 Bleeding

This is an infrequent complication reported as 0.5–2% [36]. Stopping the procedure and performing uterine massage for a few seconds usually control any serious bleeding. If not controlled with uterine massage, an intrauterine Foley catheter can be inflated with 20–30 mL of distilled water. This can be left for 12–24 h and is successful in controlling the bleeding.

12.7.3 Infection

Infection can be common post hysteroscopy but routine prophylactic antibiotics are not recommended. In prolonged procedures where the scope is introduced and removed multiple times or there is evidence of cervicitis or vaginitis, it is safer to order an intraoperative antibiotic and a course of post-operative antibiotics.

There are several reported cases of pelvic infections post hysteroscopy, and they also occur with increasing frequency in women with endometriosis [37].

12.7.4 Other Uncommon Complications Are Intrauterine Synechiae Formation

Rarely, uterine sarcomas in resected specimen have also been reported. It is therefore necessary to send all the specimens for histopathological diagnosis [38, 39].

12.8   Specific Surgical Considerations (For Prevention of Complications)

12.8.1 Hysteroscopic Myomectomy

The patient's desire to conserve uterus is to be considered, and the best possible route for surgery with the least amount of risk has to be selected. There are certain guiding principles in terms of myoma size and location. Generally a uterine size more than 16 weeks or 15 cm and individual myoma more than 6 cm are unfit for hysteroscopic removal [40, 41]. It portends a very high risk of fluid overload due to the increase in surface area of the cavity. In relation to this, any myoma occupying more than 50% the size of the cavity is unsuitable for hysteroscopic surgery. European Society for Gynecological Endoscopy (ESGE) type I myomas are best candidates for surgery. The intramural part is the biggest limiting factor in the amenability for resection. Although there are manoeuvers for making the intramural part accessible, whenever it seems bigger than estimated, the procedure should be planned in the next sitting or approached laparoscopically.

12.8.2 Hysteroscopic Synechiolysis

Synechiolysis is performed either with scissors, Colin's knife or a bipolar electrode. Intrauterine adhesions are often extensive and distort the cavity to obscure orientation. In such circumstance, marking the cornual regions with a dilator delineates the cavity, or the procedure should be performed under ultrasound guidance to prevent uterine rupture.

12.8.3 Hysteroscopic Septal Resection

Uterine septa engage the same challenges as with a synechiolysis. Determining the depth of the septa to be resected is a delicate matter. This can be determined by ultrasound or laparoscopic guidance. However in case the same is not available, the resection should generally be stopped below the inter-ostial line. Microscissors are the best tool to tackle a septum as they do not need cervical dilation or cause thermal injury to surrounding endometrium [42]. The disadvantage however is that there is also no control over bleeding.

12.9   Late Complications

Intrauterine adhesions can occur following a hysteroscopic procedure. These are rare but are known to occur following septum resection and myomectomies. Multiple strategies to reduce them have been tried, but one cannot be recommended over another with the present body of evidence. The notable interventions are intrauterine inert device placement, intrauterine balloon placement, post-operative hormone (estradiol) treatment and intrauterine instillation of anti-adhesive gel [43, 44].

Adenomyosis also is one of the complications that can result following hysteroscopic surgery. The other complication, uterine rupture, develops in a subsequent pregnancy usually after septal resection. It is more commonly associated with the use of electrosurgical devices and a history of perforation in the index surgery [45].

Conclusion/Key Points

1. Careful patient selection in terms of myoma size and location: ESGE type I myomas and size <6 cm are agreeable to hysteroscopic resection.
2. Risk stratification for cardiovascular status and kidney function evaluation before the procedure.
3. Premenopausal women are at higher risk of cerebral oedema than males or postmenopausal women.
4. Preoperative GnRH use to be considered for women with large myomas to reduce the risk of OHIS.
5. Serum Na+/K+/Cl− levels should be checked before starting the procedure and after 30 min.

6. Vasopressin infiltration reduces the risk of OHIS.
7. 1.5% glycine and 5% mannitol are solutions of choice for monopolar resection.
8. Where possible, normal saline and a bipolar source of electrosurgical generator should be used.
9. Intraoperative fluid management protocols should be observed in the theatre including the use of collecting drapes and intrauterine pressure monitoring systems.
10. In the event of occurrence of OHIS, patients should be managed with intensive support with intubation and fluid management with IV furosemide and 3% saline.

References

1. Mettler L, Patel P, Caballero R, Schollmeyer T. Hysteroscopy: an analysis of 2-years' experience. JSLS. 2002;6(3):195–7.
2. Jansen FW, Vredevoogd CB, van Ulzen K, Hermans Trimbos J. Complications of hysteroscopy: a prospective, multicenter study. Obstet Gynecol. 2000;96(2):266–70.
3. Cayuela E, Cos R, Onbargi L, et al. Complications of operative hysteroscopy. J Am Assoc Gynecol Laparosc. 1996;3(suppl 4):s6.
4. Hulka JF, Peterson HA, Phillips JM, Surrey M. Operative hysteroscopy: American Association of Gynecology membership survey. J Am Assoc Laparosc. 1995;2(1995):131–2.
5. Propst AM, Liberman RF, Hodow BL, Ginsburg ES. Complications of hysteroscopic surgery: predicting patients at risk. Obstet Gynecol. 2000;96(4):517–20.
6. Warner MA, Martin JT, Schroeder DR, Offord KP, Chute CG. Lower-extremity motor neuropathy associated with surgery performed on patients in a lithotomy position. Anesthesiology. 1994;81(1):6–12.
7. Cannì M, Gallia L, Fanzago E, Bocci F, Bertini U, Barbero M. Day-surgery operative hysteroscopy with loco-regional anesthesia. Minerva Ginecol. 2001;53(5):307–11.
8. Mushambi MC, Williamson K. Anaesthetic considerations for hysteroscopic surgery. Best Pract Res Clin Anaesthesiol. 2002;16(1):35–52.
9. Aydeniz B, Gruber IV, Schauf B, Kurek R, Meyer A, Wallwiener D. A multicenter survey of complications associated with 21,676 operative hysteroscopies. Eur J Obstet Gynecol Reprod Biol. 2002;104(2):160–4.
10. Brusco GF, Arena S, Angelini A. Use of carbon dioxide versus normal saline for diagnostic hysteroscopy. Fertil Steril. 2003;79:993–7.
11. Pellicano M, Guida M, Zullo F, Lavitola G, Cirillo D, Nappi C. Carbon dioxide versus normal saline as a uterine distension medium for diagnostic vaginoscopic hysteroscopy in infertile patients: a prospective, randomized, multicenter study. Fertil Steril. 2003;79:418–21.
12. Corson SL, Brooks PG, Soderstrom RM. Gynecologic endoscopic gas embolism. Fertil Steril. 1996;65:529–53.
13. Paull J. A prospective study of dextran-induced anaphylactoid reactions in 5745 patients. Anaesth Intensive Care. 1987;15:163–7.
14. Berg A, Sandvik L, Langebrekke A, Istre O. A randomized trial comparing monopolar electrodes using glycine 1.5% with two different types of bipolar electrodes (TCRis, Versapoint) using saline, in hysteroscopic surgery. Fertil Steril. 2009;91:1273–8.
15. Darwish AM, Hassan ZZ, Attia AM, Abdelraheem SS, Ahmed YM. Biological effects of distension media in bipolar versus monopolar resectoscopic myomectomy: a randomized trial. J Obstet Gynaecol Res. 2010;36:810–7.

16. Ayus JC, Arieff AI. Glycine-induced hypo-osmolar hyponatremia. Arch Intern Med. 1997;157:223–6.
17. Ayus JC, Wheeler JM, Arieff AI. Postoperative hyponatremic encephalopathy in menstruant women. Ann Intern Med. 1992;117:891–7.
18. Wegmüller B, Buenzli HCM, Yuen B, Maggiorini M, Rudiger A. Life-threatening laryngeal edema and hyponatremia during hysteroscopy. Crit Care Res Prac. 2011;2011:1403814 pages. https://doi.org/10.1155/2011/140381.
19. Sethi N, Chaturvedi R, Kumar K. Operative hysteroscopy intravascular absorption syndrome: a bolt from the blue. Indian J Anaesth. 2012;56(2):179–82.
20. Lee GY, In Han J, Heo HJ. Severe hypocalcemia caused by absorption of sorbitol-mannitol solution during hysteroscopy. J Korean Med Sci. 2009;24:532–4.
21. Hasham F, Garry R, Kokri MS, Mooney P. Fluid absorption during laser ablation of the endometrium in the treatment of menorrhagia. Br J Anaesth. 1992;68:151–4.
22. Garry R, Hasham F, Manhoman SK, Mooney P. The effect of pressure on fluid absorption during endometrial ablation. J Gynecol Surg. 1992;8:1–10.
23. Boyd HR, Stanley C. Sources of error when tracking irrigation fluids during hysteroscopic procedures. J Am Assoc Gynecol Laparosc. 2000;7:472–6.
24. Mavrelos D, Ben-Nagi J, Davies A, Lee C, Salim R, Jurkovic D. The value of pre-operative treatment with GnRH analogues in women with submucous fibroids: a double-blind, placebo-controlled randomized trial. Hum Reprod. 2010;25(9):2264–9.
25. Phillips DR, Nathanson HG, Milim SJ, Haselkorn JS, Khapra A, Ross PL. The effect of dilute vasopressin solution on blood loss during operative hysteroscopy: a randomized controlled trial. Obstet Gynecol. 1996;88:761–6.
26. Baskett TF, Farrell SA, Zilbert AW. Uterine fluid irrigation and absorption in hysteroscopic endometrial ablation. Obstet Gynecol. 1998;92:976–8.
27. van Dongen H, Emanuel MH, Wolterbeek R, Trimbos JB, Jansen FW. Hysteroscopic morcellator for removal of intrauterine polyps and myomas: a randomized controlled pilot study among residents in training. J Minim Invasive Gynecol. 2008;15:466–71.
28. Kumar A, Kumar A. A simple technique to reduce fluid intravasation during endometrial resection. J Am Assoc Gynecol Laparosc. 2004;11:83–5.
29. Istre O, Bjoennes J, Naess R, Hornbaek K, Forman A. Postoperative cerebral oedema after transcervical endometrial resection and uterine irrigation with 1.5% glycine. Lancet. 1994;344:1187–9.
30. Wood SM, Roberts FL. Air embolism during transcervical resection of endometrium. BMJ. 1990;300(6729):945.
31. Shaikh N, Ummunisa F. Acute management of vascular air embolism. J Emerg Trauma Shock. 2009;2(3):180–5.
32. Stankova T, Ganovska A, Stoianova M, Kovachev S. Complication of diagnostic and operative hysteroscopy- review. Akush Ginekol (Sofiia). 2015;54(8):21–7.
33. Corson SL. Hysteroscopic diagnosis and operative therapy of submucous myoma. Obstet Gynecol Clin North Am. 1995;22:739–55.
34. Howe RS. Third trimester uterine rupture following hysteroscopic uterine perforation. Obstet Gynecol. 1995;7:311–6.
35. Bellingham R. Intrauterine adhesions: hysteroscopic lysis and adjunctive methods. Aust NZ Obstet Gynaecol. 1996;36:171–4.
36. Hart R, Molnar Béla G, Magos A. Long term follow up of hysteroscopic myomectomy assessed by survival analysis. Br J Obstet Gynaecol. 1999;106:700–5.
37. Parkin DE. Fatal toxic shock syndrome following endometrial resection. Br J Obstet Gynecol. 1995;102:163–4.
38. Raiga J, Bowen J, Glowaczower E, et al. Failure factors in endometrial resection 196 cases. J Gynecol Obstet Biol Reprod (Paris). 1994;23:274–8.
39. Reed H, Callen PJ. Myometrial leiomyosarcoma following transcervical resection of the endometrium. Gynecol Endosc. 1996;5:49–50.

40. Indman PD. Hysteroscopic treatment of menorrhagia associated with uterine leiomyomas. Obstet Gynecol. 1993;81:716–20.
41. Neuwirth RS. Hysteroscopic submucous myomectomy. Obstet Gynecol Clin North Am. 1995;22:541–58.
42. Cararach M, Penella J, Ubeda A, Labastida R. Hysteroscopic incision of the septate uterus: scissors versus resectoscope. Hum Reprod. 1994;9:87–9.
43. Vercellini P, Fedele L, Arcaini L, Rognoni MT, Candiani GB. Value of intrauterine device insertion and estrogen administration after hysteroscopic metroplasty. J Reprod Med. 1989;34:447–50.
44. Abu Rafea BF, Vilos GA, Oraif AM, Power SG, Cains JH, Vilos AG. Fertility and pregnancy outcomes following resectoscopic septum division with and without intrauterine balloon stenting: a randomized pilot study. Ann Saudi Med. 2013;33:34–9.
45. Sentilhes L, Sergent F, Roman H, Verspyck E, Marpeau L. Late complications of operative hysteroscopy: predicting patients at risk of uterine rupture during subsequent pregnancy. Eur J Obstet Gynecol Reprod Biol. 2005;120(2):134–8.

Newer Developments and Future Applications of Hysteroscopy in Infertility

13

Pinky Ronak Shah

Abbreviations

ET	Embryo transfer
IVF	In vitro fertilisation
RIF	Recurrent implantation failure
RPOC	Retained products of conception
USG	Ultrasound

13.1   Introduction

The uterus plays a very important role in terms of providing adequate endometrial receptivity for implantation, further sustaining and carrying the pregnancy till term. Uterine causes contribute to 10–15% causes of infertility. Over a period of time, hysteroscopy has become vital part of Infertility workup, treating uterine causes attributing to infertility and reduction in endometrial implantation. Hysteroscopy, being simple, quick, office procedure requiring minimal anaesthesia and well tolerated by patients, over past years has become gold standard modality in diagnosing and simultaneously treating uterine pathologies. Up to 20–40% minor abnormalities are found on hysteroscopy in patients with normal transvaginal ultrasound [1]. Among all the patients who undergo pre-IVF hysteroscopy, unrecognised intrauterine pathology can be found in 18–50% of patients when there is no history of recurrent implantation failure (RIF) and in 40–43% of patients with history of RIF [2].

P. R. Shah, DGO, DNB, FNB (Reprod Med)
Morpheus Fertility Centre, Mumbai, Maharashta, India

© Springer Nature Singapore Pte Ltd. 2018
S. Jain, D. B. Inamdar (eds.), *Manual of Fertility Enhancing Hysteroscopy*,
https://doi.org/10.1007/978-981-10-8028-9_13

Hysteroscopy plays a very vital role in evaluation and treating them at the same time. Hysteroscopic endometrial scratch improves the chance of conception in patients of RIF, as induced endometrial injury is 70% more likely to result in a clinical pregnancy as opposed to no treatment [3]. Hysteroscopy has gained its popularity and is being performed worldwide in treatment of uterine causes which may contribute to infertility, prior to first IVF cycle and in patients of RIF. Considering the advantages of the procedure, hysteroscopy may have its place in new unexplored indications. Newer advances in hysteroscope and instruments and the newer applications, where hysteroscopy may prove to be beneficial, are elaborated in this chapter.

13.2   Recent Advances in Hysteroscope and Instruments

Hysteroscopy, over past years, has evolved from inpatient to a simple outpatient procedure, which is mainly attributed to more flexible, small-diameter hysteroscope. Many recent advances in the instrument have expanded the indications and also made the procedure more patient-friendly, thus providing new horizon in indications of the use of hysteroscope in the field of infertility.

13.2.1 Trophy Hysteroscope

Trophy hysteroscope is a compact, rigid hysteroscope with a diameter of 2.9 mm, 30° lens and a specially designed tip to prevent trauma. The innovative feature of this scope is the ability to load with accessory sheath in active and passive position (Fig. 13.1). Hysteroscopy can be started with single flow lumen of 2.9 mm, and in case of leakage, closure of cervical canal can be achieved by moving the accessory sheath forward, and also the view can be re-established with double flow function. The use of 5 Fr instruments is made possible in case of using the operative sheet

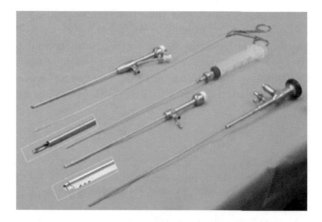

Fig. 13.1 Trophy hysteroscope with diagnostic and operative accessory sheet. Diagnostic sheet in active position providing double flow after visual controlled dilatation [Reproduced with permission: Courtesy R Campo]

Fig. 13.2 French instruments used with trophy hysteroscope [Reproduced with permission: Courtesy R Campo]

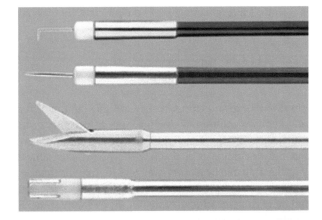

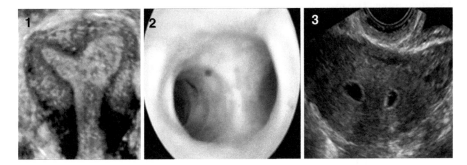

Fig. 13.3 One-stop uterine diagnosis. (1) Transvaginal sonography, (2) trophy hysteroscopy, (3) saline contrast sonography [Reproduced with permission: Courtesy R Campo]

(Fig. 13.2). This allows us to perform hysteroscopy with vagino-cervical approach without using speculum, tenaculum, anaesthesia and analgesia.

The one-stop uterine diagnosis involves performing transvaginal ultrasound followed by fluid trophy hysteroscope, immediately after which repeat ultrasound is done taking advantage of fluid in the cavity for contrast image (Fig. 13.3). If any focal endometrial pathology is seen, the trophy hysteroscope allows removing pathology with 5 Fr instruments, and interestingly curettage with trophy curette can be done without the need of speculum and also correct removal of tissue under vision.

The one-stop approach of uterine diagnosis and treatment offers advantages of having high compliance, low complication and eye-directed tissue sampling and thus opens a new dimension in screening, diagnosis and treatment of uterine pathology [4].

13.2.2 Endosee

This is handheld portable, cordless device system, which does not require anaesthesia, is well tolerated by patients and allows us to complete the diagnostic procedure in 3 min. It has advantages of no degradation of visualisation, as new camera and light source is used each time [5].

13.2.3 Virtual Hysteroscope

VirtaMedHystSim [virtual-reality training simulator for hysteroscopy] is a medical simulator for training of doctors, which trains them in diagnostic and therapeutic endoscopy. It is an excellent device for training of procedures like myomectomy and polypectomy, as it teaches the use of instruments like scissor and grasper (Fig. 13.4). It can be a promising tool to train the doctors well, giving them exposure to the hysteroscopic procedures and instruments, thus reducing complication rate and increasing the efficacy rate of the procedure. Use of original instruments for the training on the simulator eases a transfer of motor skills from simulation to the operating room. The module uses SimProctor™, a unique simulator feature guiding trainees by giving visual hints, tips and tricks to improve performance [6].

13.2.4 Firefly DE1250

This is first compact wireless digital endoscope camera with image and video capture capabilities at 30 fps. It has advantage of high magnification and light weight making it easy to use during an endoscopic procedure. The camera provides unprecedented viewing of both rigid and flexile scopes. It is a powerful tool for teaching, electronic record keeping and client communication. The software also enables users to store, view and manipulate images and video (Fig. 13.5) [7].

13.2.5 Hysteroscopic Morcellators

MyoSure: This hysteroscopic morcellator removes the target lesion by utilising electromechanical morcellation following the release of tumour by bipolar radiofrequency needle. Thus removal of FIGO or ESGE type 2 leiomyoma can be done under local anaesthesia [8].

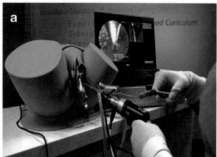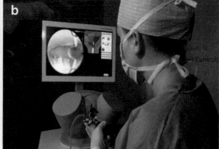

Fig. 13.4 (a, b) VirtaMedHystSim [Reproduced with permission: Courtesy VirtaMed]

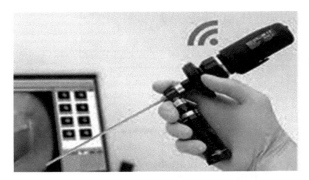
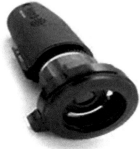

Fig. 13.5 Firefly DE1250 [Reproduced with permission: Courtesy VirtaMed]

Fig. 13.6 Standard open-sided Graves speculum (left) and Greenberg speculum (right) [Reproduced with permission: Courtesy James Greenberg]

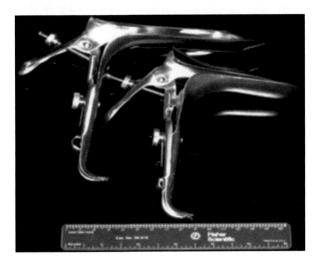

Truclear: The instrument consists of two rigid cylindrical pipes, fitted into each other, the internal acts as cutting tool, rotating within the outer at certain speed. This movement is given by an electrical control unit, which is operated by the pedal. This pedal activates and controls the direction of rotation. Both tubes have holes with cutting edges at the distal portion that cut or "shave" the tissue as it rotates, by suction continuously outward from the cavity towards a collecting container which is then sent for pathologic examination. Electrocoagulation is not used, and thus there is no risk of dispersion [9].

13.2.6 Greenberg Speculum

Greenberg speculum measures 74 mm, about 36 mm less than the standard medium-size Graves speculum. It makes insertion of hysteroscope—both flexible and rigid—easy and reduces the distance between external os and fingertips grasping the hysteroscope, by 34% or 28 mm, when compared to Graves speculum. By bringing the patient's cervix close to the operator, it reduces the length of the shaft of the hysteroscope which remains unsupported and thus yields less torque on the device entering cervical canal (Fig. 13.6) [10].

13.3   Future Applications of Hysteroscopy

Hysteroscopy may have its place in new unexplored indications, considering the advantages of the procedure. The newer applications, where hysteroscopy may prove to be beneficial, are elaborated in this chapter (Fig. 13.7).

13.3.1 Role of Hysteroscopy in IVF-Embryo Transfer

13.3.1.1   Hysteroscopic-Guided Embryo Transfer

The main contributors to success of IVF are the quality of embryos, the technique of embryo transfer and receptivity of the endometrium. Up to 30% of failed IVF cycles are due to faulty embryo transfer technique [11]. Rate of difficulty in performing the embryo transfer proportionately reduces the success of embryo transfer [12]. Any intervention that decreases difficulty of embryo transfer procedure increases pregnancy rate.

Hysteroscopic-guided embryo transfer has emerged as a new tool for patients with repeated IVF failure and history of difficult embryo transfer (Fig. 13.8).

13.3.2 Role of Hysteroscopy in History of Difficult Embryo Transfer

Difficult transfer can be caused due to tortuous and irregular cervical canal or because of acute angulation of the cervix. In the past, some measures like cervical dilatation or use of laminaria tent were performed. Also cervical canal shaving in attempt to correct the cervical cause or performing a transmyometrial transfer bypassing the cervical canal were employed. Hysteroscope can be employed as tool in patients with history of difficult embryo transfer, to normalise the tortuous cervical canal in order to avoid difficult embryo transfer in future.

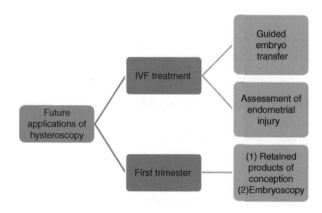

Fig. 13.7 Future applications of hysteroscopy

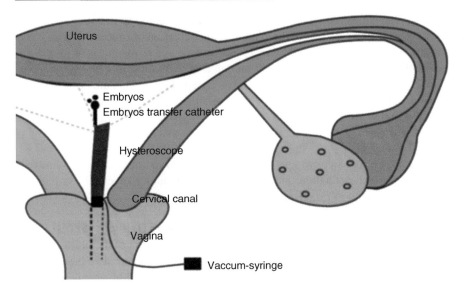

Fig. 13.8 Hysteroscopic-guided embryo transfer

In a case series of 36 patients with history of difficult intrauterine procedures because of tortuosity or stenosis of cervical canal, endocervix was evaluated and corrected hysteroscopically. It was followed by transcervical placement of a male-cot catheter. Thirty-two out of 36 patients had significantly easier procedures after the procedure. Correction of endocervical abnormalities may lead to improved pregnancy rates after IVF-ET, as the ease of embryo transfer has been correlated with improved implantation rates [13]. In the future, hysteroscopy can be a promising tool in such patients and can be a replacement of difficult transmyometrial transfers.

13.3.3   Hysteroscopic-Guided Embryo Transfer in Patients with Previous Failed IVF Cycles

In patients with repeated failed IVF-ET attempts, hysteroscopic-guided embryo transfer can be utilised to increase clinical pregnancy rates. The embryos are deposited on to the endometrium under direct vision. Kilani et al. performed the procedure by inserting 5 mm hysteroscope, avoiding cervical dilatation, and using CO_2 as distension medium. CO_2 is delivered at constant flow using hysteroflator at 100 mL/min until internal os was seen. They avoided passage of hysteroscope beyond internal os to prevent any endometrial damage or bleeding. Embryos were loaded on the embryo transfer (Wallace) catheter. The soft catheter was introduced in the operating sheath after being withdrawn from rigid sheath, and embryos were deposited 1 cm below fundus. A successful live birth was reported by authors [14].

In another study on **hysteroscopic endometrial embryo delivery (HEED)**, Kamarva et al. reported two to three times higher chances of conception than blind transfer technique. Using flexible mini hysteroscope and nitrogen gas as distension media, the embryos were transferred on day 2 or 3 by a flexible embryo transfer catheter. The proposed benefits of HEED as reported by authors are correct placement of embryos at the desired site in a minimal volume of media, hence less chances of retained embryos and lower ectopic pregnancy rate. The disadvantage of the procedure is the additional cost, invasive nature and risk of disruption of endometrial lining [15].

The role of hysteroscopy in performing guided embryo transfers looks promising and needs further evaluation and more randomised studies especially in patients with previous failed IVF cycles.

13.3.3.1   Hysteroscopic Subendometrial Embryo Delivery [SEED]

The process of implantation involves apposition and adhesion of the blastocyst followed by invasion of endometrium. The concept of subendometrial embryo transfer is based on the hypothesis that the blastocyst when inserted mechanically under vision into the endometrium may enhance the success rate of IVF.

Subendometrial blastocyst transfer under hysteroscopic guidance was performed by Kamarva et al. The procedure utilised 3 mm flexible mini hysteroscope. The distension of the endometrial cavity was achieved by the nitrogen gas (50 cm^3 at 70 mmHg) to allow the movement of scope in gaseous space and to avoid contact with endometrium, thus reducing any endometrial trauma by the instrument itself. The embryos were deposited under direct hysteroscopic vision, by semi-rigid catheter, at a depth of 1 mm into endometrium. There were five clinical pregnancies out of 15 IVF cycles [16]. The advantages of SEED include:

(a) Direct visualisation of the cavity and deposition of embryos at different sites if there is inadvertent trauma
(b) Reduced chances of uterine contractions as it prevents the catheter tip touching the fundus
(c) Loading of embryos in lesser amount of media, thus decreasing the risk of ectopic pregnancies

The potential drawbacks of the procedure are scratching of endometrium, invasive nature and cost. Further prospective, controlled and randomised studies are required to confirm the role of hysteroscopic subendometrial transfer in IVF cycles.

13.3.3.2   Role of Hysteroscopy in Assessment of Endometrial Integrity and Damage Caused by Embryo Transfer Catheter

Factors affecting the success of the embryo transfer procedure are blood on the catheter, uterine contractions, catheter type, catheter loading, catheter tip placement, use of trial transfers and pre-transfer ultrasound [17]. Embryo transfer under ultrasound guidance allows clinician to deposit the embryos in the endometrial cavity, avoiding touching the fundus, which can initiate uterine contractions and decrease the pregnancy rate. Little have been surveyed on effect of embryo transfer catheter on endometrial integrity, which is very essential for successful implantation. Hysteroscope is a promising tool, taking a step forward, and provides more information on relation of difficulty associated with the procedure and its impact on endometrial integrity and extent of damage to the endometrium.

Murray et al. assessed endometrial damage following mock embryo transfer by hysteroscopy. In patients who had easy embryo transfer, there was no endometrial damage in 54% and moderate to severe damage in 37%. No clear association was found in the amount of endometrial damage and difficulty of transfer, in patients who had moderate difficulty in the embryo transfer procedure.

The authors concluded clinical perception of ease of transfer does not correlate well with the degree of endometrial disruption ($p = 0.41$), thus highlighting the lack of accuracy in scoring transfers clinically. The authors observed certain endometrial defects, like non-bleeding furrows and focal subendometrial haemorrhage, were due to catheter used for transfer, and thus they proposed the use of hysteroscopy to assess differences between catheter types. Further, it can be used as training tool for clinicians, helping them develop their ET techniques and achieve excellence in this rate-limiting step, avoiding excessive endometrial damage and thus improving IVF outcome [18].

More randomised trials are required to provide information on damage to endometrium by soft or rigid catheters and relation of the ease of procedure and effect on endometrium.

13.3.4 Role of Hysteroscopy in First Trimester

13.3.4.1 Role of Hysteroscopy in Removal of Retained Products of Conception and Preservation of Fertility

Retained products can lead to an inflammatory response in the endometrium causing formation of adhesion. A blind curettage technique for removal of products of conception can cause trauma to basalis layer, leading to formation of adhesions, which may affect the future fertility. The risk of developing intrauterine adhesion after curettage performed for miscarriage is around 66.7% [19]. Hysteroscopy allows direct visualisation and complete removal of retained products and thus can reduce risk of adhesions and repeat interventions.

A meta-analysis and literature review on hysteroscopic removal of products of conception concluded that hysteroscopy is superior to traditional curettage and has low complication rates (uterine perforation, infection and vaginal bleeding), low rates of intrauterine adhesions (5.7%) and high rates of subsequent pregnancies (75%) [20]. It is associated with shorter time to conceive and lower rate of newly found infertility problems, when compared to traditional dilatation and curettage [21].

13.3.4.2 Embryoscopy

First-trimester miscarriages are seen in around 15–20% of pregnancies, and approximately 60–70% of these miscarriages are secondary to detectable chromosomal abnormalities [22]. Hysteroscopy when performed after confirmation of pregnancy failure in first trimester is called embryoscopy. Embryoscopy allows directed biopsy which avoids contamination with maternal tissue or blood found on samples that are collected by suction and evacuation, and thus it improves cytogenetic testing. Though chromosomal abnormalities are often the cause of missed abortions, other defects involved can be screened for by transcervical embryoscopy.

Although it is possible to introduce mini endoscope transcervically to observe the early embryo, the optical resolution has not been satisfactory. Rigid mini endoscope can now be introduced transabdominally and transmyometrially to observe the embryo in situ with better resolution.

Philipp et al. performed transcervical embryoscopy prior to dilatation and curettage, on 272 patients diagnosed with missed abortion. On cytogenetic analysis of chorionic villi, authors found abnormal karyotype in 75% of patients, morphological defects in 18% of patients with normal karyotype and no chromosomal or embryonic abnormality in 7% of patients.

In patients with history of repeated pregnancy losses, this correlation between morphological defects on embryoscopy and cytogenetic findings in abortion specimens provides information to the physician regarding genetic counselling about risk of recurrence and antenatal care in future pregnancies [23].

In future, hysteroscopy can be aid in search for diagnosis of first-trimester abortions and simultaneously avoiding risk of uterine adhesions.

13.3.5 Future Scope of Research to Evaluate Newer Applications of Hysteroscopy

There are still many unexplored indications of hysteroscopy, which may be studied in future expanding newer applications of hysteroscopy.

Hysteroscopy can be employed in performing intrauterine insemination, depositing washed semen sample near the cornual end, towards the side of patent tube in patients of unilateral tubal block. It can be combined with endometrial receptivity assay so that patients of recurrent implantation failures can undergo two procedures simultaneously. Both procedures can help the practitioner to establish the cause of RIF, counsel the patient and formulate plan of treatment. A novel role of hysteroscopy can be explored in first trimester when β HCG is positive, but below discriminatory zone and ultrasound is inconclusive. Office hysteroscopy can play a role in helping to make a decision of putting in laparoscope in selective symptomatic patients. Hysteroscopy can be used as a tool in instillation of endometrial stem cell therapy, thus providing hope to patients who are not willing for surrogacy and may replace need of uterine transplantation (Fig. 13.9).

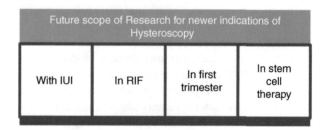

Fig. 13.9 Future scope of research for newer indications of hysteroscopy

Conclusion

The role of hysteroscopy as primary assessment in infertile couples is well established. It is found to be efficacious in diagnosis and simultaneously treatment of intrauterine defects. The scope can further be expanded in procedures like hysteroscopic-guided embryo transfer and embryoscopy and in patients who had difficulty in embryo transfer procedures once adequate evidence becomes available. Ongoing interventions in smaller-diameter scopes, newer developments in various designed hysteroscopes, instruments and equipments and associated optical devices have expanded the horizon of its indications and therapeutic benefits in infertile couple. Newer advances in hysteroscope and simulators will enable clinicians to gain proficiency and confidence in many hysteroscopic-guided unexplored procedures, before attempting them on patients. Combination of newer tools and advanced technology will expand its role in infertility, and thus the future of hysteroscopy looks promising!

References

1. Koskas M, Mergui JL, Yazbeck C, Uzan S, Nizard J. Office hysteroscopy for infertility: a. series of 557 consecutive cases. Obstet Gynecol Int. 2010;2010:168096. https://doi.org/10.1155/2010/168096.
2. Bozdag G, Aksan G, Esinler I, Yarali H. What is the role of office hysteroscopy in women with failed IVF cycles? Reprod Biomed Online. 2008;17(3):410–5.
3. Potdar N, Gelbaya T, Nardo LG. Endometrial injury to overcome recurrent embryo implantation failure: a systematic review and meta-analysis. Reprod Biomed Online. 2012;25(6):561–71.
4. Campo R, Meier R, Dhont N, Mestdagh G, Ombelet W. Implementation of hysteroscopy in an infertility clinic: the one-stop uterine diagnosis and treatment. Facts Views Vis Obgyn. 2014;6(4):235–9.
5. www.endosee.com. Assessed on 12 Mar, 2017.
6. https://virtamed.com/hystsim. Assessed on 30 May 2017.
7. www.fireflyglobal.com. Assessed on 31 May 2017.
8. Munro MG. Hysteroscopic myomectomy of FIGO type 2 leiomyomas under local anesthesia: bipolar radiofrequency needle–based release followed by electromechanical morcellation. J Minim Invasive Gynecol. 2016;23(1):12–3.
9. www.intervalolibre.wordpress.com. Assessed on 12 Mar, 2017.
10. Greenberg JA. The greenberg hysteroscopy speculum: a new instrument for hysteroscopy. JSLS. 2006;10:129–13.
11. Cohen J. How to avoid multiple pregnancies in assisted reproduction. Hum Reprod. 1998;13(suppl 3):197–214.
12. Spandorfer SD, Goldstein J, Navarro J, Veeck L, Davis OK, Rosenwaks Z. Difficult embryo transfer has a negative impact on the outcome of in vitro fertilization. Fertil Steril. 2003;79(3):654–5.
13. Yanushpolsky EH, Ginsburg ES, Fox JH, Stewart EA. Transcervical placement of a Malecot catheter after hysteroscopic evaluation provides for easier entry into the endometrial cavity for women with histories of difficult intrauterine inseminations and/or embryo transfers: a prospective case series. Fertil Steril. 2000;73(2):402–5.
14. Kilani Z, Shaban M, Hassan LH. Live birth after hysteroscopic-guided embryo transfer: a case report. Fertil Steril. 2009;91(6):2733.e1–2.
15. Kamrava M, Tran L. Hysteroscopic endometrial embryo delivery (HEED). In: Kamrava M, editor. Ectopic pregnancy- modern diagnosis and management. Rijeka, Croatia: In Tech; 2011. p. 79–86.

16. Kamrava M, Yin M. Hysteroscopic sub endometrial embryo delivery (SEED), mechanical embryo implantation. Int J Fertil Steril. 2010;4(1):29–34.
17. Schoolcraft WB, Surrey ES, Gardner DK. Embryo transfer: techniques and variables affecting success. Fertil Steril. 2001;76:863–71.
18. Murray AS, Healy DL, Rombauts L. Embryo transfer: hysteroscopic assessment of transfer catheter effects on the endometrium. Reprod Biomed Online. 2003;7(5):583–6.
19. Schenker JG, Margalioth EJ. Intrauterine adhesions: an updated appraisal. Fertil Steril. 1982;11:593–61.
20. Smorgick N, Barel O, Fuchs N, Ben-Ami I, Pansky M, Vaknin Z. Hysteroscopic management of retained products of conception: meta-analysis and literature review. Eur J Obstet Gynecol Reprod Biol. 2013;173:19–22.
21. Ben-Ami I, Melcer Y, Smorgick N, Schneider D, Pansky M, Halperin R. A comparison of reproductive outcomes following hysteroscopic management versus dilatation and curettage of retained products of conception. Int J Gynaecol Obstet. 2014;127(1):86–9.
22. Tariverdian G, Paul M. Genetic aspects of disorders in early pregnancy. In:Genetic diagnosis in obstetrics and gynaecology, Guidelines for clinic and practice. Berlin: Springer publishing house; 1999. p. 191–8. https://doi.org/10.1007/978-3-642-58453-4.
23. Philipp T, Philipp K, Reiner A, Beer F, Kalousek DK. Embryoscopic and cytogenetic analysis of 233 missed abortions: factors involved in the pathogenesis of developmental defects of early failed pregnancies. Hum Reprod. 2003;18(8):1724–32.